HYANNIS PUBLIC LIB
ASSOCIATION
W9-BEF-209

Celiac Disease

Celiac Disease

A Guide to Living with Gluten Intolerance

Sylvia Llewelyn Bower, RN

with

Mary Kay Sharrett, MS, RD, LD, CNSD
Steve Plogsted, PharmD

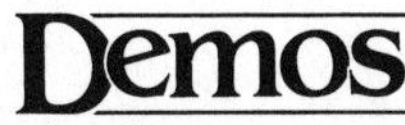

616.399

Visit our website at www.demosmedpub.com

© 2007 by Demos Medical Publishing, LLC. All rights reserved. This book is protected by copyright. No part of it may be reproduced, stored in a retrieval system, or transmitted in any form or by any means, electronic, mechanical, photocopying, recording, or otherwise, without the prior written permission of the publisher.

Library of Congress Cataloging-in-Publication Data
Bower, Sylvia Llewelyn.
Celiac disease : a guide to living with gluten intolerance / Sylvia Llewelyn Bower with Mary Kay Sharrett, Steve Plogsted.
p. cm.
Includes bibliographical references and index.
ISBN-13: 978-1-932603-25-5
ISBN-10: 1-932603-25-5
1. Celiac disease—Popular works. 2. Gluten-free diet—Popular works.
I. Sharrett, Mary Kay. II. Plogsted, Steve. III. Title.
RC862.C44B69 2006
616.3'99—dc22

2006006035

The purpose of this book is to provide a basic overview of living with celiac disease, some examples of how others have dealt with the condition, and some guidelines to assist in everyday living. It should not be construed as medical advice. Readers should always consult with their doctors.

Special discounts on bulk quantities of Demos Medical Publishing books are available to corporations, professional associations, pharmaceutical companies, health care organizations, and other qualifying groups. For details, please contact:

Special Sales Department
Demos Medical Publishing
386 Park Avenue South, Suite 301
New York, NY 10016
Phone: 800-532-8663, 212-683-0072
Fax: 212-683-0118
Email: orderdept@demosmedpub.com

Made in the United States of America
06 07 08 09 10 5 4 3 2 1

This book is dedicated to my sister, Betty Elmquist, who gave continued encouragement and editing while it was being written, and to my Lord who gave me the faith that it could be accomplished.

Special thanks to the many members of the Gluten-Free Gang who shared their stories and experiences in their daily walk as a celiac or as parents of a celiac.

And to my family, which has provided love and support to me from the time of my diagnosis of celiac disease.

Contents

Preface

The purpose of this book is to give peace of mind to individuals diagnosed with celiac disease (CD). Knowledge will set them free. Family members and health care professionals both can gain insight and information to guide and encourage newly diagnosed individuals.

Each chapter was written to inform, challenge, and encourage the individual with CD. It is a personal disease that affects many different body systems and continues to have many unanswered questions regarding:

- factors that trigger CD;
- factors that prevent CD;
- the relationship between CD and autoimmune disorders;
- the health economic consequences of CD.

The medical profession has taken giant steps in its ability to diagnosis and treat CD. Even as recently as 1997, CD was considered an extremely *rare* disorder. Occasionally, a biopsy of the patient's small intestine, preceded by numerous long-term symptoms, made a diagnosis possible. Physicians have made an impact on the amount of accumulated research over the past three to five years.

Individuals living with CD are always interested in research because the more information our physicians have, the more comprehensive the treatment can be.

Many researchers and physicians across the United States and Europe have created projects and written papers contributing to the increased knowledge.

Two prominent physicians contributing to the research are Dr. Joseph Murray from the University of Iowa, who is now continuing his research at the Mayo Clinic, and Dr. Allesio Fasano, from Italy, where CD is prevalent. Dr. Fasano started the Celiac Research Center at the University of Maryland, and was instrumental in a United States study that challenged the International Gastroenterologists to more actively research CD. Dr. Peter Green has done research in his practice at Columbia Presbyterian in New York. The University of Chicago and Stanford are also active in research. There are also more researchers across this country, as well as in Europe.

Celiac disease is considered to be the most underdiagnosed common disease, with an average length of time of 11 years between onset of symptoms and confirmation of diagnosis.

A large multicenter study of over 13,000 children and adults in the United States has found that CD is far more common than previously thought and reported. The details of this study can be found in the February 10, 2004, issue of *Archives of Internal Medicine*. According to their findings, there are about 2 million Americans with CD.

The incidence of CD in families with CD is 1:22 for first-degree relatives (parents and siblings), 1:39 in second-degree relatives (grandparents, aunts, uncles, and cousins), and 1:56 in symptomatic patients.

The American Celiac Disease Alliance includes representatives from all of the research centers, celiac organizations, and published literature. They are working with the U.S. Congress and the Federal Food and Drug Administration (FDA) to lobby for improved food labeling.

Most recently, the National Institutes of Health sponsored a Consensus Panel that challenged the medical community to recognize the prevalence of CD. Data from this panel is used throughout the book.

We have written this book with the hope that the information it provides will make a "new" celiac's journey easier.

Sylvia Llewelyn Bower
Mary Kay Sharrett
Steve Plogsted

CHAPTER 1

What Is Celiac Disease?

Courage is the first of human qualities because it is the quality which guarantees all the others.

—Winston Churchill

Celiac disease (CD) has gone from the depths of the darkest pits of ignorance into the light of knowledge within the last 5 years. "For wisdom will enter your heart and knowledge will be pleasant to your soul," according to Proverbs 2:10. Knowing all about CD will empower you to discuss it, share your information and experiences, teach about it and, above all, live with it!

No expensive pills, elixirs, lotions, or injections can heal the body of a person with CD. Understanding CD and following a strict diet are the only ways that people with CD can eliminate their symptoms. After being diagnosed, it is possible to regain your health, even though no medication is available to cure the disease. A lifelong diet that excludes wheat, barley, and rye and all their derivatives is the only option for treatment. Each person is responsible for following the diet and ultimately eliminating the symptoms. However, it is dangerous to go on a gluten-free diet before you have been diagnosed, because then a diagnosis cannot be made.

Pathology of CD

Celiac disease is defined as a multisystem disorder that causes the body's immune system to respond to the protein in certain grains. The immune system builds antibodies against these proteins and causes damage to the small intestine. The wheat-type grains have protein complexes called *gliadin* that are harmful to people with CD. The barley-type grains have protein complexes called *hordein*, and rye has protein complexes called *secalin*. The chemical make-up of the gliadin, hordein, and secalin cause the body to have an immune reaction. It is still not understood why these grains do this. Gluten is found in other grains, such as corn, yet it causes no ill effects to CD patients.

The harmful forms of gluten are found in these grains and grain-derived products:

- Barley
- Couscous
- Kamut
- Malt
- Matzo
- Rye
- Semolina
- Soy sauce
- Spelt
- Sprouted barley
- Sprouted wheat
- Teriyaki sauce (unless wheat free)
- Triticale
- Udon
- Wheat

This list also includes all regular baking flours, breads, pasta, pastries, and desserts made with the above flours.

An antibody test evaluates if *endomysial antibodies* are present in the blood. The autoantigen for the endomysial antibodies is the enzyme *tissue transglutaminase*. This has led to an assay that uses either guinea-pig or human (tTG) tissue transglutaminase to identify CD.

The individual must have a genetic predisposition to activate CD. According to Dr. Peter Green, of Columbia University, 98% of people with CD share the genes identified as HLA-DQ2 and HLA-DQ8. He states that "People who do not have HLA-DQ2 or HLA-DQ8 haplotypes are unlikely to have coeliac disease." It is possible to have symptoms and, if a genetic test is run and these haplotypes are not present, still not fit the diagnosis of CD.

In the digestive process, chewed food, mixed with saliva, goes from the mouth, into the esophagus, and enters the stomach, where gastric juices mix with the food. The food continues to travel into the small intestine. Nutrition from the food is absorbed through small projections, called villi, on the surface of the small intestine. The villi absorb the nutrition from the digesting food.

In CD, the gluten in certain grains causes the body to produce endomysial antibodies. These antibodies create an inflammatory process that destroys the villi (Figure 1-1). Previously, this destruction was thought to be gluten-sensitive enteropathy, gluten intolerance, or even possibly a wheat allergy. The most recent information from the University of Chicago indicates that only CD causes villi destruction. The other conditions do not.

CD was, until the last few years, thought to be very rare in the United States. Few physicians realized its potential impact or researched its prevalence. Dr. Alessio Fasano, who came from Italy to the University of Maryland, reasoned that if 1 in 150 in Italy are prone to CD, then the United States, with its large European heritage, should have a high prevalence. This research suggests that 1 in 133 persons in the United States are at risk for CD. This would suggest that approximately 2 million U.S. residents have CD. The research indicates that the worldwide prevalence is 1 in 250.

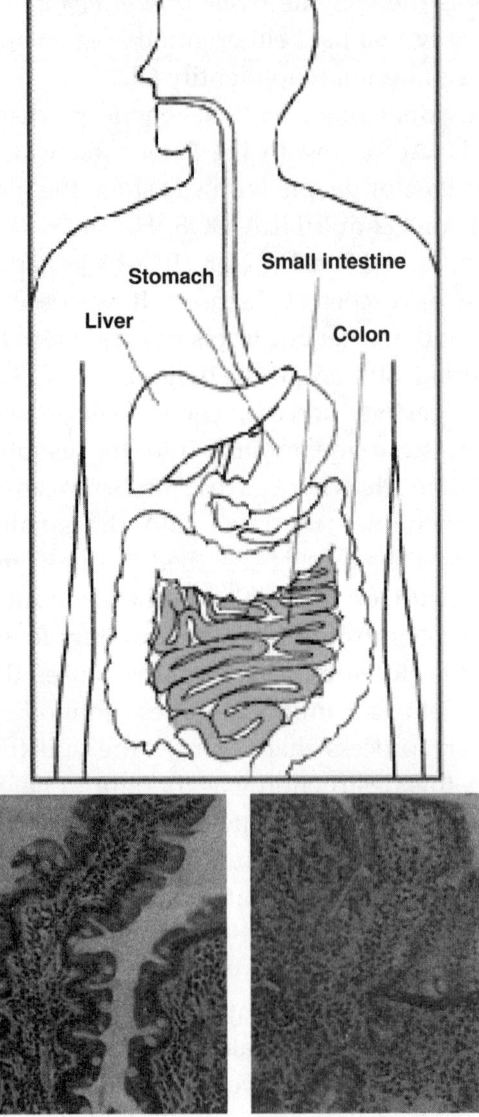

Figure 1-1. (Top) The digestive system. (Reprinted from *Celiac Disease*, from the National Digestive Diseases Information Clearing House, National Institute of Diabetes & Digestive & Kidney Diseases, National Institutes of Health.) (Bottom) On the left is a normal villi which has indentations to absorbs nutrients. On the right, the fingerlike projections are gone and the surface is basically flat and would have difficulty absorbing nutrients. (This image was used by permission by the Department of Pathology of the University of Kansas.)

> Celiac disease is isolating, and the isolation can hurt far more than the treatment. Suddenly, you find yourself on one side of a fence, the sick side. Everyone else in your world is on the other side of that fence—the normal side.

Obviously, if absorption is disturbed, nutrients from food will not enter the body. The food will continue to pass through the large intestine and be eliminated. The entire body may show symptoms because it is not receiving enough fuel to function.

The age of onset varies from infancy to the elderly, and the symptoms can be very subtle or obvious. However, one commonality exists for each individual diagnosed with this disease: No one is sure what triggers the disease. Some statistics show pregnancy, a virus, or stress may be the trigger, but no clear cause is obvious.

An infant may show symptoms when he is introduced to grains at an early age. The symptoms may include diarrhea, constipation, foul-smelling stools, fatigue, slow growth pattern, irritability, and even a swollen belly from malnutrition. An older adult frequently presents with anemia from no apparent cause.

It is not known why one person may develop CD at 6 months and another doesn't show symptoms until they are in their Golden Years. The average age of diagnosis, based on statistics, is between 40 and 60.

Symptoms

The symptoms of CD may be varied and hard to define. The individual with CD may know she "feels bad" and realize that something is wrong, but be unaware of what to do about it. One of the most familiar presentations of the disease is that the patient will feel tired and listless. If it persists, the doctor will usually order a blood test.

The most common result of such testing is iron-deficiency anemia. This anemia is caused by the body not absorbing iron from the food that is eaten. In CD, the damage to the intestine may be so great that iron cannot be absorbed, and it is then possible that other nutrients, such as calcium and protein, also are not being properly absorbed.

Dr. Peter Green states that: "Celiac disease is a very common disorder, and most people with the disease have the silent form. These individuals are usually identified through screening of at-risk groups."

Because of the variety of symptoms presented, the disease is often overlooked by physicians in this age of the medical specialist. A patient may consult a psychiatrist, psychologist, or mental health social work for symptoms of irritability, depression, and behavior changes. An orthopedic specialist or rheumatologist may be consulted for joint pain, bone pain, or osteoporosis. A dentist will see the individual for symptoms of dental enamel hypoplasia and sores in the mouth, but be unaware of his patient's other physical symptoms. An allergist may discover lactose intolerance or an allergy to milk or wheat. A dermatologist may be asked to treat the painful itching skin rash but, unless the skin is biopsied for dermatitis herpetiformis, CD will go undiagnosed because doctors do not usually associate diet with skin rashes.

One form of CD causes very itchy, scaly skin lesions. When the skin is biopsied, CD can be identified through the antibodies present. This is called *dermatitis herpetiformis,* and it also causes the intestinal damage described in Figure 1-1.

A hematologist may find that the person suffers from anemia of unknown origin. A neurologist will treat seizures or unsteady walking (ataxia), but may not be able to discover a clear reason for the episode because the patient's electroencephalogram does not show brain lesions.

The family practitioner will have on file the symptoms of abdominal pain, bloating, constipation, diarrhea, chronic fatigue, and gas. However, if the physician is not familiar with CD, the referral to a gastroenterologist, which should be the first step toward a correct diagnosis, might not be made.

It is easy to see how the medical community might diagnose this individual as a hypochondriac. Many with CD have traveled from doctor to doctor, seeking relief from single symptoms when, if the pieces of the CD puzzle were only put together, their problem could be diagnosed easily.

According to Ann Whalen of *Gluten-free Living* and The National Institutes of Health (NIH) the following individuals should be tested for CD:

- Those with classic symptoms of chronic diarrhea, malabsorption, weight loss, abdominal distention
- Those with short stature, delayed puberty, iron-deficiency anemia, recurrent fetal loss, infertility
- Those with irritable bowel syndrome, persistent aphthous stomatitis (cold sores), autoimmune diseases, peripheral neuropathy, cerebellar ataxia, dental enamel hypoplasia

Populations at risk include individuals with type I diabetes mellitus, first- and second-degree relatives of individuals with CD, individuals with Turner syndrome, and those with Down or Williams syndromes.

CHAPTER 2

Diagnosis

Success is to be measured not so much by the position that one has reached in life as by the obstacles which he has overcome while trying to succeed.

—Booker T. Washington.

People with celiac disease (CD) can suffer with symptoms for years before being diagnosed. The key to better health is automatically turned when a diagnosis is rendered. However, the key opens the door to a healthy lifestyle only if a gluten-free diet (GFD) is maintained. Adhering to the diet reduces the risk of complications.

The typical individual with CD may go to many doctors before being diagnosed. Sometimes it is necessary for a person suffering with abdominal bloating, pain, diarrhea, and/or constipation to rule out other diseases. Some of the problems that should be ruled out are irritable bowel syndrome, Crohn's disease, ulcerative colitis, diverticulitis, intestinal infection, chronic fatigue syndrome, and possibly other conditions not associated with the intestinal tract.

The first step to a diagnosis begins with a laboratory test. Continue to eat gluten until tested. If you go gluten-free, the protein that causes the antibodies will not be present to indicate CD, even if you have it.

Your blood will be tested for the presence of IgA tissue transglutaminase (tTG) and immunoglobulin

A antiendomysium (AEA) antibodies. These tests are considered 98% accurate and specific for CD.

If your blood tests are positive, it is recommended that your physician follow-up with an endoscopy, in which a biopsy is done to identify the extent of damage to the small intestine. This test is done on an outpatient basis. A flexible tube is introduced through the stomach and into the small intestine. A mild sedative is usually given as part of this procedure. The endoscopy allows a gastroenterologist to examine the intestine and take a biopsy. The specimen is then sent to the laboratory to verify the diagnosis. (A new technology for this is called the *wireless capsule endoscopy.* A miniaturized camera is swallowed and the remote camera visualizes the intestine. The problem with this procedure is that, if the villi are flat, then a regular endoscopy still must be done for the biopsy.)

Once the diagnosis is obtained, the challenge of managing the disease begins. Following a GFD for life is now the standard treatment. If gluten is ingested, the intestinal villi, as explained in Chapter One, are destroyed. By eating gluten-free foods, the villi are not challenged or irritated by the gluten protein, and so are allowed to heal. This does take time. The first few months may cause some anxious moments if you think you've eaten something that contains gluten.

After diagnosis, it will take a few weeks, or even months, to start feeling an improvement in your health. The amount of irritation CD has wrought on your body varies, as does the time required for the healing process. Do not be discouraged. Stay on the GFD. (Some research suggests that the age at diagnosis determines how long it takes to heal, but this has not been confirmed.)

If you are not be feeling well and wondering why, you may have to re-evaluate your diet to make sure you're not eating anything—vitamin pills, candies, medicines, or foods—that may contain gluten.

(You may also be diagnosed with lactose intolerance, which further complicates your diet. See Chapter Three for important information on this condition.)

Early Diagnosis Is Important

Take a proactive role in your health problems. Ask your physician to order the necessary tests to rule out other possibilities. The importance of physicians diagnosing CD within the early stages was discussed in an article published by Leffler, Saha, and Farrell in *The Managed Care Journal.* It states that early diagnosis can prevent many of the complications associated with the disease. If you continue to have symptoms, and you've been unsuccessful in obtaining a clear diagnosis, take this book or a copy of the bibliography in the back of this book, to your physician and ask him to consider the possibility that you may have CD.

For physicians as well as for patients, the learning curve at this juncture is difficult. Even though the amount of knowledge available is increasing, many health professionals are still unaware of the disease.

The more you know about CD, the easier it will be to make the adjustment to living a gluten-free lifestyle. Educating family and friends with adequate information will also make sure that meals are prepared and served gluten-free. Some family members may not understand your special dietary needs, and it may be necessary to take food with you when you visit, or invite them to sample a gluten-free meal. It may take months of educating, but eventually most people will understand that you must follow a very strict diet, and they will be glad to help you. It may be helpful if you can compare your dietary restrictions to those who have other diet-related disorders, such as diabetes or food allergies.

Sherry gives a great personal testimony of her experience with CD diagnosis:

"The symptom that eventually led my doctors to a diagnosis of celiac disease is not a classic symptom of the condition. The swallowing trouble I began having at age 39 was an atypical symptom and puzzled my doctors and me for 4 years. After several noninvasive tests that were negative for any causes of swallowing problems (e.g., cancer), my doctors concluded that anxiety might be the cause.

"Not convinced, I underwent both an endoscopy and esophageal manometry, which revealed the muscles were not functioning normally. The question that remained unanswered for the next 4 years was Why?

"After a few years of eating soft foods which, ironically, were high gluten-containing foods like pasta and taking antacids, I pressed my gastroenterologist for more testing. During the second endoscopy, a biopsy tested positive for *sprue* (which is another name for celiac disease). I will always remember my doctor saying, "Don't worry" and reassuring me that I could not possibly have this because it was too rare! But, because the test was positive, he ordered blood work, which confirmed the surprising diagnosis. I finally had some answers about why I was anemic, why I lost so much weight, and why I had trouble eating!

"Since CD was considered rare at the time (I was diagnosed in 1993), the first dietitian I went to admitted that she would have to learn along with me. Luckily, she had some familiarity with gluten-free foods to recommend to me, and she also sent for diet information from the Gluten Intolerance Group of America.

"After months of struggling to make sense of all the new and sometimes conflicting information about the diet, I learned about our support group in Columbus. I was excited to learn about the annual celiac conferences organized by clinical dietitian, Mary Kay Sharrett and Dr. B. Li of Children's Hospital, both of whom had special interests in supporting and educating celiac patients. What a relief it was to get the guidance I needed to follow a GF diet, and support other celiacs to help me meet all the challenges that sometimes seemed overwhelming."

At the onset of the disease, it is not uncommon to have insatiable cravings, apparently caused by anemia, nausea, or abdominal pain. A member of the Gluten-Free Gang Support Group, submitted the following as an example of initial symptoms:

More Ice Cubes, Please!

"I had crunched ice most of my life, but never like this. When I was pregnant with my second child, I would go through the ice from our automatic icemaker so fast that I bought four extra ice cube trays to freeze each day to keep up with my "demand." When that supply was exhausted, I would beg my husband to go buy me a 10-pound bag of ice. This was a sign of anemia caused by my undiagnosed celiac disease. I was severely anemic, experiencing extreme fatigue, heart palpitations, and shortness of breath. I had no gastrointestinal symptoms or weight loss. My due date was approaching and, to ensure a safe delivery, I was given a blood transfusion and multiple intravenous iron infusions. In the end, the doctors (my OBGYN and hematologist) concluded that the anemia had been caused by the pregnancy.

"About 1 month after the baby was born, I suddenly began having severe diarrhea. At first, I assumed that I had eaten a bad hamburger at a fast food restaurant the day before it started. However, the diarrhea would not go away. I called my doctor who, after informing me that viruses were going around, prescribed an antidiarrheal medication. It did help a little bit with the symptoms, but I was still afraid to leave my house (and my bathroom). After complaining to the doctor a few more times, he decided to test my stool for infectious organisms. The results were negative.

"I had a feeling that my problems were due to more than just a virus. I called the doctor one more time, and he did the best thing he could have done. He referred me to a gastroenterologist. After a colonoscopy, an upper endoscopy, and a simple blood test, it was confirmed that I had celiac sprue disease, 5 months after my initial bout with diarrhea had appeared.

"I have been on the gluten-free diet for a little over a year, and I am happy to say that the ice cubes in my freezer are going stale for the first time that I can ever remember.

Living with CD

The ultimate way to start living with CD is to ask for a care conference that includes your doctor, dietitian, family, pharmacist, registered nurse and a member of a CD support group. This is the ideal way to obtain valuable information, provide the best continuity of care, and achieve the best optimum outcome. Within the medical profession, many complicated problems are approached using this method, so you are justified in asking for this.

CARE CONFERENCE

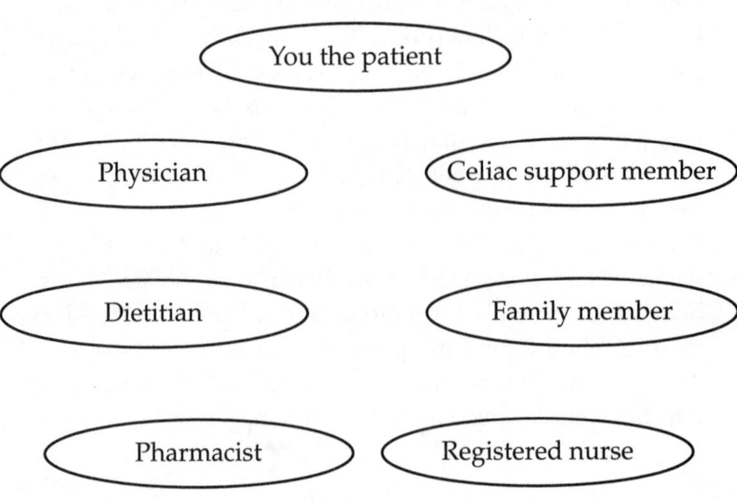

The professionals participating in a care conference represent different disciplines. Each will present information about his particular aspect of the disease and how it effects you. Your general physician will be aware of your total medical condition, prescription medications you are taking, and the results of the testing that you have had, and he may wish to share a plan for specific follow up. Your dietitian will be able to make recommendations for dietary changes and offer resources regarding food supply and educational opportunities. A registered nurse may be asked to coordinate all disciplines, acting as your patient advocate, and to assist in creating a plan of care for you. Your family members will gain a better understanding of the challenges, genetic predisposition, common symptoms, and the necessity of a lifelong diet in CD. Finally, your pharmacist can evaluate all your medications to see if they contain gluten.

Your individual needs can be best met through this multidisciplinary approach. It is the most effective way for all disciplines to understand what approach will work best to get you on the road to recovery.

If you cannot assemble a care team, then make individual contacts on a one-to-one basis. It is most important to meet with a dietitian familiar with CD to determine the list of foods allowed and where to obtain them.

Remember, being in charge of your diet is the most important thing that you do. You are still a person with all your strengths and abilities. The disease has nothing to do with that. By taking control, you can remain confident and have the assurance of living a healthy life. Sherry summarized her story with a remarkable ending. "The GF diet consists of many healthy foods and includes a surprising variety of alternative grains. I am grateful to have answers to many life-long problems and thankful that I have a condition that can be treated through dietary modification. What continues to motivate me is the commitment to better health and desire to set a good example for my adult children."

CHAPTER 3

Dermatitis Herpetiformis

Life is a pure flame, and we live by an invisible sun within us.
—Thomas Browne

Dermatitis herpetiformis is a chronic eruption of the skin characterized by clusters of intensely itchy, small bubbles and allergy- or hive-like lesions that are slow to heal (Figure 3-1). The disease is usually found in patients 30–40 years old and is more common in men than in women. It occurs rarely in African Americans and Asians. All normal appearing skin will have antibody (IgA) deposits. The rash, which is caused by an allergic reaction to gluten, is often called "celiac disease of the skin."

The herpes virus does not cause DH, even though the name suggests it. Herpetiformis means "grouped vessels" and describes the rash that accompanies DH. The rash is often confused with other kinds of allergic skin rashes. As mentioned above, the actual cause is the body's response to the gluten protein found in wheat, barley, and rye. Allergies like hives are usually caused by the IgE antibodies of the immune system. DH is caused by the IgA antibody, which is produced in the lining of the intestine. The usual forms of allergy treatments are not effective in treating DH.

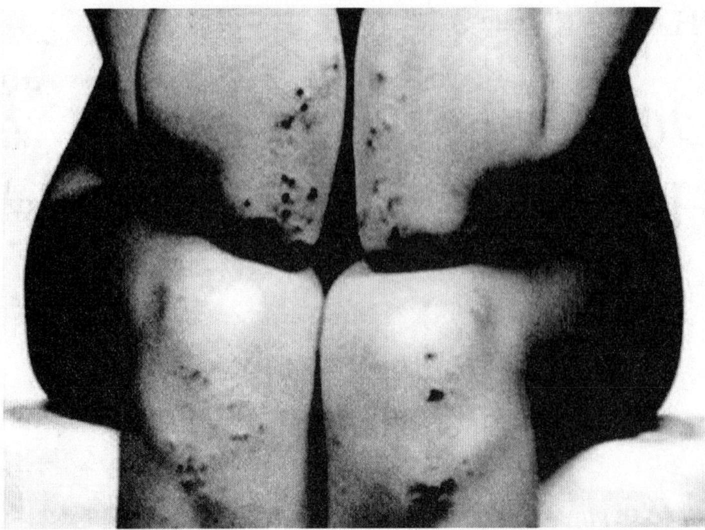

Figure 3-1. An example of dermatitis herpetiformis (Used by permission of the University of Chicago Celiac Research Center).

When the gut is affected by the inflammatory response to the proteins in wheat, barley, and rye so that the villi are inflamed and/or destroyed, it is called gluten-sensitive enteropathy (GSE), or celiac disease. Some people with DH do not have GSE and others do. Because there are cases of GSE that have turned cancerous (malignant lymphoma), an evaluation by a gastroenterologist is important. It is interesting that the signs and symptoms of malabsorption in DH are usually absent, and there is no association between the intensity of the intestinal damage found at biopsy of the small intestine and the intensity of the skin lesions in DH. GSE is found in 75%–90% of DH patients, indicating that they are directly connected to CD.

Dr Stefano Guandalini from the University of Chicago Celiac Disease Program recently wrote an article for the "DX: Celiac" newsletter which he has agreed to allow us to include here. The article is one of the most recent and comprehensive statements about DH, and the authors thank him for his permission to use it.

Dermatitis herpetiformis (DH) is a condition that raises many questions and concerns among parents and patients, ranging from how to distinguish an allergic skin reaction from actual DH to the optimal management of DH once diagnosed.

DH is an uncommon skin manifestation of celiac disease, affecting mostly adults. It has a prevalence of approximately 1–2 in 10,000 people. DH is characterized by the appearance of small pimples and blisters, typically on the elbows. They may also appear on the knees, face, scalp, trunk, buttocks, and occasionally within the mouth. The lesions are symmetrically diffused. The predominant symptoms are itching and burning that is rapidly relieved when the blisters rupture.

The earliest abnormality is a small reddish spot about one-eighth of an inch in diameter that quickly develops into a "bump." Small blisters then appear and tend to merge together. Scratching causes them to rupture, dry up, and leave an area of darker color and scarring.

As DH is not common, usually the diagnosis takes a long time. The dermatologist will confirm DH by obtaining a skin biopsy (best if taken at the edge of the lesion, not on the affected skin). The pathology exam of the biopsy will show the typical deposition of granular immunoglobulin A (IgA)in the skin by a microscopic exam with a method called immunofluorescence. The disease is in fact thought to result from an aggression of IgA autoantibodies directed against the skin-associated tissue transglutaminase.

What makes DH unique is its association with celiac disease. In fact, DH is celiac disease: they share exactly the same genetic background (DQ2 and/or DQ8), each condition is more frequent in families where the other is also found, they are both triggered by an autoimmune response to gluten, and they are associated with other autoimmune conditions such as thyroiditis (found in as many as 1 in 4 DH patients.)

DH and CD also are characterized by the same type of gluten-induced damage to the intestinal mucosa (the flattening of the villi) and they both carry an increased risk—when not treated—of lymphomas.

Thus, if DH is diagnosed, celiac disease is also present and the same strict gluten-free diet must be started.

Dr. Guandalini also describes the differences between DH and CD:

- The predominance of females vs. males in CD is reversed: DH is found twice as frequently in males;
- The mean age of onset is later in DH, around 40 years, with childhood DH being a rare occurrence;
- There is a higher prevalence (about 20%) of serologically negative (tissue transglutaminase and/or endomysial antibodies negative) patients with DH; therefore serological screening in DH is not as effective as it is in celiac disease.
- Signs and symptoms of malabsorption in DH are usually absent or minor.
- There is no association between the intensity of the intestinal damage found at biopsy of the small intestine and the intensity of the skin lesions in DH.

He goes on to say:

> Because of the typical gastrointestinal problems and the slow response (months to years) to a strict gluten-free diet (GFD), some patients with DH think they have no benefit from the diet and do not follow it, relying only on the pharmacological treatment with Dapsone. *This is a mistake!* Dapsone will suppress, but not cure the disease, and is completely ineffective on the intestinal lesion: on the other hand, GFD results in clearing of the skin disease and of the intestinal damage. To further support this concept, reintroduction of gluten has been found to result in the recurrence of the disease (within weeks).

> Correctly treating this disorder and preventing its complications, requires the daily use of oral Dapsone (that relieves the itching within 2 days) and an ongoing, strict GFD. Dapsone is tapered off as time on the gluten-free diet lengthens, and Dapsone should eventually be discontinued."

Continuing on a strict gluten-free diet is still considered the best treatment for CD and DH. Both conditions are genetic and both cause destruction in the small intestine. The frustration that occurs with DH is that it can take a long time for the lesions to clear after going gluten-free.

There has always been a question as to whether topical items such as shampoo, lotions, and other skin products need to be gluten-free for the celiac. Dr. Peter Green in his new book *Celiac Disease: A Hidden Epidemic* states "that unless you are eating these products, they are not going to cause a DH flare-up."

Bob, a professional man, came to the Gluten-Free Gang when he was first diagnosed with DH. He has agreed to give us his story and experiences with DH.

> It was not long after I developed a very itchy rash on my elbows, forearms, knees, and sacrum in late 2000 that I made an appointment with a dermatologist to have it checked out. The itch was so intense it pretty much consumed my everyday life and was more severe than I was accustomed to experiencing with poison ivy on numerous occasions throughout my life. Attempts at using topical creams to alleviate the itch were, for the most part, futile. I probably suffered through it for about three months until I sought medical help. Although the first dermatologist noted I exhibited the classic findings of dermatitis herpetiformis (DH), the initial skin biopsy proved to be taken improperly, which resulted in negative immunofluorescense results. A follow-up punch biopsy by another dermatologist a few months later proved to be successful and I was clinically diagnosed with DH.

During the interim between both biopsies, I was prescribed Dapsone to see if it would alleviate the rash. It literally only took about 2 to 3 hours for the intense itching to completely subside. Although the rash was still present and took longer to somewhat clear up, it was a relief the itch abated and I was able to get a full night's sleep. The dermatologist mentioned I was probably only the second case of DH he's ever diagnosed and that the disease was due to having wheat in my diet. That's all I was told as I walked out his door.

I had no idea what the rash really entailed until I researched it on my own through Internet searches and discovered it was closely associated with an incurable condition called celiac disease and that the only lifetime treatment for it was the adherence to a gluten-free diet. Unlike a classic celiac patient, I had no gastrointestinal symptoms such as cramping, diarrhea, or constipation. The only indication that I suffered intestinal damage was a history (at least 5 years) of anemia. I also learned that some environmental/stressful factor or body trauma likely triggers the disease to begin manifesting itself. In my case, it may have been attributed to a surgery I had in July 1998.

I was pretty overwhelmed after learning all the foods I was no longer able to eat. At the time of my diagnosis, I was 30 years old, athletic, and very active. I had (and still maintain) a high metabolism and was always eating. I relied heavily on carbohydrates, particularly for breakfast and snacks. I realized I needed some counseling to help me with the dietary change. To just suddenly give up certain foods, particularly breads, desserts, pasta, and beer was quite a sacrifice—especially my mom's Hungarian cooking and pastries! Through the Internet, I contacted the Gluten Intolerance Group in Seattle, and was referred to a Central Ohio dietitian, Mary Kay Sharrett, who dealt closely with celiac patients and served as a liaison for a local support group called the Gluten-Free Gang. My initial anxiety about trying to adhere to a gluten-free diet was alleviated after I met with Mary Kay for diet instruction and began attending the group meetings for tips and guidance.

Through time, I gradually adjusted to the change in my diet and was able to adapt by substituting certain foods for what I used to consume. I had to learn to accept that I might never be able to taste the foods I grew up with my entire life—there was no turning back. I have to admit, I am a pretty dedicated person and will stick to a regime if it is for my well-being. I was never a finicky eater. I ate just about anything, anytime, that was put in front of me. I was challenged all the time, particularly when I had to leave my comfort zone at home and travel for work, typically every 6 weeks, most of the time to San Diego or the San Francisco Bay areas. I was lucky in this respect and couldn't have asked for better destinations. California was famous for its abundance of heath-food stores and seafood and Mexican cuisines. However, I also traveled to remote places in West Virginia as well as in the Deep South, where just about everything is fried. No matter where my travels took me, once arriving at my destination, I would immediately go grocery shopping, particularly for breakfast and lunch items. I always stayed in hotel rooms equipped with a fridge and microwave at a minimum. If small kitchens were available, I requested those rooms. During the workday, I always packed my lunch and abundant snacks in a small cooler. On numerous occasions when eating out with co-workers when we were travelling, I would usually agree to the consensus of where to eat without knowing the menu. It was too embarrassing and complicated trying to explain my restricted diet to everyone, and there was no way I was going to rain on their parade with the wide choice of cuisines that San Diego and the Bay Area offered. Because I was not a finicky eater, there was always sometime I could eat, even if it meant having just a salad at an Italian restaurant to hold me over until I got back to my stash in the hotel room. With time, my close friends and co-workers became understanding of my diet and were willing at times to compromise their choice of cuisine for my sake.

At home, my wife was also trying to deal with the dietary change. I would usually kid her that it was pretty coincidental that my DH/celiac disease manifested soon after we got married. I never expected her to surrender her diet to accommodate mine. In actuality, I only had to tailor my diet slightly to adapt to what we made in the past. We always maintained a healthy diet. We rarely ate fast food, frozen dinners, or prepared fried foods. I had my own cupboard with my own pastas, flours, mixes, etc. I picked up on a good sourdough recipe for bread through the GFG and bake my own buns for sandwiches. The only specialty foods I purchase from health food stores are gluten-free cereals, pancake mixes, pastas, crackers, and the occasional brownie mix. I really never had a sweet tooth so only once in a blue moon do I buy GF cookies and cakes.

However, I was still coping with the rash flare-ups associated with DH. Even though I started omitting gluten from my diet, there was still an abundance of antibodies in my body from all the gluten I ingested in the past. I learned that it commonly took 5 to 7 years until the body was rid of the antibodies that caused the skin disorder. Wow, I thought—7 years of an intense constant itch that I had to try to maintain with the Dapsone. Even though the Dapsone alleviated the itch most of the time, the rash would still erupt spontaneously, resulting in constant scratching that opened sores and caused them to bleed, soiling my clothes, our linens, furniture, etc. After the sores scabbed up, they, too, warranted scratching because they were typically located on joints that were subjected to constant stretching and irritation. It was embarrassing in public because there was no way I could not scratch some part of my body, which usually led to bleeding. If I had a penny for every time my wife chastised me for scratching in public, I would have more than enough money to buy those heavily priced gluten-free beers by the case. She just assumed I popped a pill (Dapsone) and my troubles would be over.

As the years went on, I had blood tests performed quarterly to determine, first, whether my antibody count was decreasing and second, to make sure the Dapsone was not damaging my liver, thus enabling me to get refills. The serological testing was the only way I could gauge whether my diet was working. If I accidentally ingested gluten, which I have done at times on the GF diet, there was no way of knowing it. I was still getting the rash no matter what. With no rhyme or reason, the rash seemed to make it to just about every part of my body at some point.

Looking back, it is almost as if it would erupt pretty fiercely for 6 months to a year at one location before phasing out and going on to another body part. The rash would eventually develop on my scalp and the back of my neck (resulting in embarrassing trips to the barber), my eyebrows, underarms, elbows, forearms, wrists, scapula (most difficult part to scratch), hips, sacrum, buttocks, knees, calves, shins, and currently on my ankles and feet. Many times I wished I had the gastrointestinal symptoms because at least they manifested very soon after a mishap and I could deduce what foods I consumed had gluten. Then I got to thinking: If I screwed up and accidentally ingested gluten at some point during the diet, did that 7-year clock reset itself from that point on? It was a very frustrating time. I tried to limit the dosage of Dapsone I took and only increased it when a rash erupted. Gradually, to my relief, the diet began to kick in, enabling me to decrease my dosage. Serological tests showed non-detectable levels of antibodies. My rashes were not really erupting anymore but rather coming on slowly with minimal itching sensations.

Currently, after six years, I would have to say my body is about 95 percent gluten free. I do not think I will ever reach 100 percent, but it is to a stage where I am no longer taking Dapsone, but rather have it handy in case of an "episode."

I never travel without it. I have learned that because my body is pretty much free of antibodies, when I do accidentally ingest gluten, it takes about 10 days to two weeks for the rash to erupt (but who knows where on my body it will decide to show up) and last only about a month or two before clearing up. I still have minor rashes, but nothing compared to a full-blown eruption that would have me popping a Dapsone.

As a result of having full-blown DH for 6 years, I have developed a scratching habit, whether it is warranted or not, and almost as a nervous habit. My body is riddled with scars from constantly scratching the same scabs off numerous times, and (to my wife's relief) I am not doing laundry as much as I used to. Finally, I have to say that, at 38 years old, I am in the best health I have ever been.

A very honest testimony from Bob, who has been through it.

CHAPTER 4

A Healthy Gluten-Free Diet

by Mary Kay Sharrett

We shall steer safely through every storm, so long as our heart is right, our intention fervent, our courage steadfast, and our trust fixed on God.

—St. Francis De Sales

A gluten-free diet (GFD) is the only treatment for celiac disease (CD). Therefore, making sure your food is gluten-free is key to staying healthy. However, you must do a few other things to make your diet both gluten-free *and* healthy. Some concern exists that the GFD may be low in B vitamins, iron, calcium, and fiber; if it took several years for you to be diagnosed with CD, then you were not absorbing some of these same nutrients very well. Most gluten-free grain products are not enriched or fortified with B vitamins and iron, as their gluten-containing counterparts are required to be. Also, some people with CD are diagnosed as being lactose intolerant; because they have trouble tolerating milk, they decrease or eliminate milk and milk-containing products from their diets, thus making their diets deficient in calcium and vitamin D. In addition, many gluten-free products are based on corn, potato, and rice starches and so have very little fiber. Therefore, it is not only important to learn what foods are gluten-free, but also to learn what foods to include in your diet to stay healthy.

Making It Gluten-Free

The first step in living with CD is learning what foods are gluten-free. The GFD eliminates all foods prepared with wheat, rye, oats, barley, and their derivatives. The elimination of oats has been controversial for years. Several recent studies have indicated that oats, in moderate amounts ($1/2$ cup), may be safe for adults and children with CD. However, the cross-contamination of oats with other gluten-containing grains during the harvesting and milling process is a concern. The elimination of wheat starch has also been controversial; wheat starch is allowed in some foreign countries although, just like oats, some concern exists that the wheat starch available in the United States is contaminated with gluten. Therefore, wheat starch and oats should be eliminated from your diet until an acceptable source can be found.

Many gluten-free grains and vegetables (some new to American diets) are good sources of vitamins, minerals, protein, and fiber. The following grains and/or starches are gluten-free:

- Amaranth
- Arrowroot
- Bean
- Bean flour
- Buckwheat
- Corn
- Flax
- Indian rice grass
- Legumes
- Lentils
- Mesquite
- Millet
- Montina
- Nuts
- Potato
- Quinoa
- Rice
- Sorghum
- Soy
- Tapioca
- Teff
- Wild rice

However, all these grains and starches may become contaminated during the milling and manufacturing process, so it is important to purchase them from manufacturers who take precautions to eliminate cross-contamination.

All food labels must be carefully examined to determine product contents. (Table 4-1 lists ingredients to avoid.) If an ingredient is questionable, the food manufacturer must be contacted for more information. Table 4-2 contains a list of ingredients you should check on. Gluten can lurk in almost anything you ingest. Even medications may contain gluten, so a knowledgeable pharmacist or physician should examine all prescribed and over-the-counter medications for gluten content. Products such as toothpaste and mouthwash also need to be gluten-free. If you are in

Table 4-1. Ingredients to avoid on a gluten-free diet

Wheat	**Triticale**	**Malt, malt flavoring, malt syrup**	**Bulgur**
Rye	Spelt (dingus)	Graham flour	Wheat gluten
Oats	Kamut	Graham crackers	Orzo
Barley	Flour	Wheat germ	Farina
Semolina	Cereal	Seitan	Wheat starch
Durham	Farro	Matzo, matzo meal	Cracked wheat
Emmer	Einkorn	Malt vinegar	Couscous

Table 4-2. Ingredients to question

Modified food starch
Caramel coloring*
Flavorings
Dextrin*
Soy sauce
Brown rice syrup (May be made from barley)
Starch in medications

*Caramel coloring and dextrin are currently not being made with gluten-containing ingredients.

doubt about a product, it is best to avoid it until you can thoroughly investigate it!

Become an avid label reader. Food manufacturers do have the option to change their ingredients, and the labels are changing. A new labeling law called the Food Allergen Labeling and Consumer Protection Act (Public Law 108–282) was passed in the summer of 2004. This new law requires food manufacturers to declare the source of ingredients when they contain one of the top eight allergens (milk, eggs, peanuts, tree nuts, fish, crustacean shellfish, soy, and wheat). Barley and rye are not considered one of the top eight allergens, but many manufacturers are including them in their labeling changes.

Make It Nutritious

A healthy GFD should include a wide variety of foods. For the majority of adults and children, your diet should include 2 to 4 servings of fruits, 3 to 5 servings of vegetables, 6 to 11 servings of gluten-free grains, and 3 to 4 servings from the milk food group. Making wise choices from all of these food groups can help provide the nutrients that are of concern in the GFD.

Enriched? Fortified?

Enriched and fortified mean that a food has nutrients (usually vitamins and minerals) added to it to make it more nutritious. *Enriched* is defined as adding back nutrients that were lost during the processing of the product. *Fortified* means adding nutrients that are not present in the original product. In the 1940s, the U.S. Food and Drug Administration (FDA) developed standards for refined white flour. Their original goal was to add the thiamine, niacin, and riboflavin (the B vitamins) lost during the processing of wheat. Since then, the FDA has required the addition of iron and folic acid. They have also made provisions for the optional addition of calcium. These standards were developed because of concern that American diets were deficient in these nutrients. Gluten-free grain products are not required to be enriched and fortified. However, many foods allowable in the GFD, especially fruits, vegetables, and legumes, are good sources of these nutrients (Table 4-3). Canada recently made provisions that gluten-free grain products should be enriched and fortified with the same amount of nutrients as their gluten-containing counterparts. Some enriched and fortified gluten-free products are available, and there are plans for many more.

Fiber

The new Dietary Reference Intakes (DRIs) recommend that Americans increase their intake of fiber because it can help prevent and treat many different health-related issues such as obesity, cardiovascular disease, type 2 diabetes, and constipation. The DRI for children 1 to 3 years is 19 grams of fiber per day; for children 4 to 6 years, 25 grams per day; for teenage boys, 31 grams per day; for teenage girls 26 grams per day; for men age 19 to 50 years, 38 grams and age 51 and older, 31 grams; for women 19 to 50 years 25 grams and age 51 and older, 21 grams. Yet the average American only eats 11 grams of fiber per day.

Constipation, rising cholesterol levels, and weight control problems are common issues among CD patients following a GFD. (See Table 4-4 for are some suggestions to increase your fiber intake.) You can find out how much fiber is in your diet by looking at the Nutrient Facts Label on your food. Remember to look at the serving size, too. If you are not eating enough fiber, gradually add more to your diet—but do it slowly, because a large increase in your fiber intake at one time may cause you some abdominal discomfort and gas.

Table 4-3. Food sources of nutrients

Iron	**Folate**	**Thiamin**
Best sources: Pork loin, sardines, molasses, oysters, clams *Good sources:* Lean beef, kidney beans, spinach, shrimp, pinto beans, greens, tuna, navy beans, avocado, dried apricots, tempeh (soy product), lentils, raisins, potatoes with skin, green peas, lima beans, prunes, figs	Liver and other organ meats, eggs, spinach, pineapple, tomato juice, asparagus, corn, bananas	*Good sources:* Beef liver, pork (lean), enriched corn tortilla, enriched rice *Fair sources:* Cantaloupe, honeydew, orange juice, watermelon, corn, peas dry beans, lentils, pine nuts, sunflower seeds
Riboflavin	**Niacin**	**Vitamin B_{12}**
Good sources: Beef liver, yogurt, milk, enriched corn tortilla, egg *Fair sources:* Broccoli, mushrooms, spinach, sweet potato, almonds	*Good sources:* Turkey, peanut butter, enriched corn tortilla, Codfish, black-eyed peas, lima beans	Organ meats (beef and lamb liver, kidney, heart), clams, oysters, nonfat dry milk, crabs, salmon, sardines, rock fish, egg yolk

Table 4-4. Tips for increasing your fiber intake

Add kidney beans, garbanzos, or other bean varieties into your salads. Each half-cup serving contains approximately 7 to 8 grams of fiber.
Use whole-grain flour when possible in your cooking and baking, and choose whole-grain bread. Some gluten-free flours that are high in fiber are buckwheat, amaranth, quinoa, corn meal, garbanzo flour (chickpea), garfava flour (garbanzo and fava bean), and montina.
Add rice bran or corn bran to recipes or use as a topping on gluten-free cereals or yogurt. Corn bran has 4 grams of fiber per tablespoon, and rice has 1.5 grams of fiber per tablespoon. Gluten-free rice bran is available from Ener-G, Bob's Red Mill, El Peto, Glutino, and Kinnickkinnick. Gluten-free corn bran is available from Glutino.
Some commercial fiber supplements are gluten-free. Benefiber made from guar gum has 3 grams of fiber per tablespoon. Benefiber is made by Novartis and is available in some local grocery stores.
Eat at least five servings each day of fruits and vegetables. Juices don't have fiber. Fresh fruit has a slightly higher fiber content than canned. While all fruits have some fiber, some are higher than others. A few that have 3 to 4 grams of fiber per serving include apples, pears, 1 cup of blueberries, 1 cup of strawberries, oranges, and tangerine. Raspberries are high in fiber, with 8 grams per cup. Vegetables can be good sources of fiber also. Those that have 3 to 4 grams of fiber include: 1/2-cup squash, 1/2-cup peas, 1 cup carrots, 1/2-cup cauliflower, and 1 medium sweet potato.
Add chopped dried fruits to your cookies, muffins, pancakes, or breads before baking. Dried fruits have a higher amount of fiber than the fresh version. For example, 1 cup of grapes has about 1 gram of fiber, but 1 cup of raisins has almost 7 grams. Packaged fruit leathers or snacks have no fiber.
Nuts and seeds are excellent sources of fiber (avoid offering to children under age 4 who may choke on these). A 1/4 cup of the following nuts and seeds contain 3 to 4 grams of fiber: sunflower seeds, peanuts, sesame seeds, and almonds.

Continued

Table 4-4. (Continued)

Add flax. Flax is a great source of fiber and other nutrients. Flax seed must be broken up in order for you to absorb nutrients and benefit from the fiber Use a coffee grinder to grind the seed, and grind as you need it. You can store whole flax seed at room temperature. Store ground flax in the refrigerator or freezer. Add it to cereals and yogurts.

Cook with brown rice rather than white rice. If it's hard to make the switch, mix them together. One cup of brown rice is $3\frac{1}{2}$ grams of fiber. Wild rice is also a good source of fiber—1 cup has 9 grams of fiber.

Choose fiber-rich snacks such as popcorn (1 gram of fiber per cup), raw vegetables with reduced-fat dip, rice bran crackers with cheese, and trail mix.

Lactose Intolerance

Lactose is the natural sugar found in milk. *Lactase* is the enzyme that digests lactose, and it is found on the tips of the villi in the small intestine. If your intestinal villi are damaged, then you may not be producing enough lactase. When lactose is undigested, it travels through the intestine and gets digested and used by the normal bacteria that reside there. This bacterial activity can cause gas and pain; it also attracts water to the intestine and usually results in diarrhea. Thirty to sixty percent of adults diagnosed with CD also have lactose intolerance. Very few children have lactose intolerance at diagnosis.

The treatment for lactose intolerance in conjunction with CD is a GFD and a temporary reduced-lactose diet. Once your intestine heals, you should be able to tolerate lactose, although some may never able to tolerate lactose. If you have to follow a lactose-restricted diet, you must eliminate milk and products made with milk such as ice cream, cottage cheese, and some other cheeses. However, these foods provide you with calcium and vitamin D, which are very important to your bone health. Many adults and children have low bone mineral density or even osteoporosis at diagnosis because they have not been absorbing calcium and vitamin D very well. Therefore, to maintain bone health, adequate intakes of calcium and vitamin D are important for newly diagnosed CD patients, as well as for everyone with CD.

If you have lactose intolerance, try to include milk that has been treated with an enzyme such as Lactaid. Aged cheese has very little lactose in it, and yogurt with active enzyme is usually well tolerated. You can also take an enzyme with your meals that will break down the lactose before it reaches the small intestine. Another tip is to eat lactose-containing foods with a meal, rather than between meals. If you still can not tolerate 3 to 4 servings from the milk group, make sure you work with your dietitian to get the proper amounts of calcium and vitamin D supplements. (Gluten-free supplements are listed in the Appendix and on the website www.glutenfreedrugs.com.)

Vitamins and Minerals

An age-appropriate multivitamin with minerals is recommended for people with CD. However, taking a multivitamin is not a substitute for good eating habits. Food provides an ideal mixture of essential nutrients that cannot be captured in a pill. Therefore, taking recommended amounts of vitamins and eating a healthy diet is recommended. Taking large doses of some vitamins or minerals can cause deficiencies of other vitamins or minerals, so be sure to work with your dietitian and doctor if you are taking more than the recommended amounts of vitamins and minerals. (Gluten-free vitamins and minerals can be found listed in the Appendix and on the Web at www.glutenfreedrugs.com.)

CHAPTER 5

Complications

The world will never starve for want of wonders.
—Gilbert Keith Chesterton

Most research recognizes celiac disease (CD) as a multisystem disorder. This means that it can have an effect on many different body systems. It was originally thought that the only organ involved in CD was the small intestine. However, just as the pieces of a puzzle are assembled, as more research is completed, a number of other conditions have been found associated with CD. For example, researchers at Cornell University and the Minneapolis VA Hospital have recognized that neuropathy and several other neurologic syndromes are associated with CD, and that these present as extraintestinal symptoms.

Dental enamel defects also are prevalent in celiacs. By realizing that this results from calcium malabsorption, it is indicated that bone deficiencies and dental enamel defects could be caused by a complex syndrome that prevents normal bone formation. A gluten-free diet (GFD) is the only recommendation for treatment until further studies can be done. In addition, many children go to their doctors with unrelated symptoms, such as growth failure, malabsorption, and unstable diabetes; many pediatricians are now suggesting that all type I diabetic children be screened for CD.

A fine line can be drawn between the symptoms caused by CD itself and by the complications of the disease. The state of being unable to absorb nutrients through the small intestine because of the result of damage *is* CD. In addition, however, it has been proven that, in CD, the small intestine becomes permeable and gluten is able to pass through its walls, thus causing the complications that lead to other systemic conditions. We'll examine the known complications of CD in the sections of this chapter.

Known Complications of CD

Inflammation

As CD progresses, it causes inflammation of the small intestine. The tissue of the small intestine weakens, becomes reddened, and the texture actually changes. This permits fluid and gluten to pass through the small-intestinal wall into the abdominal cavity and be absorbed by the circulation of the blood. This is known as a *permeable gut* condition and it leads to problems. The body only functions in a healthy manner as long as everything stays where it belongs.

Anemia

Anemia in people with CD is thought to be the result of the small intestine's inability to absorb iron. When the body does not absorb iron, not enough blood cells are created to carry oxygen. This causes the individual to experience extreme fatigue. Every part of the body suffers when it does not receive enough oxygen.

Calcium Malabsorption

When the body cannot absorb calcium, the bones become porous and prone to osteoporosis. A person with osteoporosis may suffer from multiple broken bones. Without calcium, the texture and density of the bones actually changes. If permitted to progress, the slightest impact or even an abrupt motion, can cause damage to the bones. Also, this same mechanism is considered to be the cause of dental enamel deficiencies.

Cancer

One of the most immediate concerns of all persons with CD is their increased chances of acquiring one of three different types of cancer: non-Hodgkins lymphoma, esophageal cancer, and adenocarcinoma of the small intestine. These cancers may be caused by the constant irritation and chronic inflammation of the small intestine's mucosa or lining. When a CD patient is diagnosed and adheres to a GFD, the risk of developing adenocarcinoma and esophageal cancer drastically decreases. The risk of non-Hodgkins lymphoma does not decrease, according to some of the research. (Some things in life we cannot control and, since research shows that mental attitudes do affect our health, this is the time for you to live life to the maximum in a gluten-free state.)

Infertility and Pregnancy

When a woman is having reproductive problems, such as conceiving a child, carrying a pregnancy to term, or experiencing menopausal upheavals, she should ask her doctor to evaluate her for CD. When the body is not in sync because of CD, nothing works right.

Undiagnosed women with CD have a high rate of miscarriage. If a pregnancy is carried to term, an infant can be born with neural tubal defects caused by the lack of absorption of folic acid. Many women have gone on a GFD and delivered normal healthy babies. It is suggested that a

CD mother breast-feed as long as possible because it has been recognized that breast feeding delays the appearance of CD.

Menopause

The undiagnosed CD woman has a heavy burden to carry during menopause. By not having a diagnosis, the woman is dealing with celiac symptoms as well as menopausal symptoms. The GFD can help to balance some of the body's mechanisms while hormone levels are changing.

Neurologic Symptoms

Recent research on CD and neurologic disorders suggests that between 10% and 51% of CD patients may exhibit signs of neurologic symptoms, as opposed to 19% of the general population without CD. The wide disparity between these two numbers may be accounted for by different methods in how the research was conducted and where the research was done; recognized symptoms of CD may differ, depending on where the diagnosis is made. Research on CD is only starting, and all research results give us more parts of the puzzle that will eventually fit together to make a big picture.

In one study, about 10% of people with CD were diagnosed as having the following neurologic disorders:

- Ataxia (disturbance of walking balance)
- Attention deficit disorder
- Depression and/or anxiety (common in about 20% of CD patients)
- Neuropathy (the loss of nerve function)
- Seizure disorders

Other neurologic researchers claim that the following symptoms are found in 51% of all CD patients, compared with 19% in the non-CD population:

* Attention deficit hyperactivity disorder (ADHD)
* Cerebellar ataxia (disturbance of walking balance)
* Developmental delays (children slow in speech and coordination)
* Headaches
* Learning disorders

It is important to note that these neurologic symptoms should never be brushed off simply as part of CD. Each symptom must be evaluated by an appropriate specialist. A neurologist should evaluate seizures and ataxia, while a psychiatrist should evaluate depression, anxiety, and attention deficit disorders. Neuropathy is a common symptom of diabetes.

Depression

The newest literature shows that depression is common among people with CD and that a GFD sometimes helps depression. Some people may need medication to balance the brain's chemistry, while others may need counseling. The important issue is to take control of one's destiny. A person with CD must be aggressive concerning improving all aspects of her life, including physical, psychological, and spiritual well-being.

Diabetes

Many children visit their doctor with unrelated symptoms, such as growth concerns, malabsorption, or unstable diabetes. It is recommended by some physicians that all diabetic children be screened for CD.

Dermatitis Herpetiformis (see Chapter 3)

It is a fact that 25% of CD patients have a skin condition called dermatitis herpetiformis. This condition can be biopsied and help to diagnose CD. The skin eruptions are extremely itchy and are a manifestation of the damage that is happening in the small intestine. These skin symptoms improve on a GFD. Dermatitis herpetiformis is a form of CD, and actually not a complication.

Suspected Complications of CD

Other known conditions that may be complications of CD are still in the research stage. These could be considered suspected complications.

Liver Disorders

Several liver disorders have been identified with CD, such as:

- Increased liver enzyme levels
- Nonspecific hepatitis
- Nonalcoholic fatty liver disease
- Cholestatic liver disease

Cholestatic liver disease is the most common liver disorder among CD patients. This disease occurs when the bile duct from the gall bladder to the liver is suppressed, and the bile does not flow.

Other Observed Conditions

Other conditions frequently seen with CD include:

- Fibromyalgia (pain in the fibrous areas of muscles)
- Aphthous ulcers (sores in the soft mucous membrane of the mouth and tongue)

* Joint pain
* Down syndrome (It is estimated that 20% of all individuals with this condition have CD)
* Dysrhythmia (an abnormal heart rate)
* Autoimmune diseases (CD is identified as an autoimmune disease)
    * Lupus erythematosus
    * Insulin dependent diabetes
    * Autoimmune thyroid disease
* Multiple sclerosis
* Sjögren syndrome

Genetics and CD

The genetic factor in the CD puzzle cannot be ignored. If an individual has CD, there is a 90% chance of them having the gene that has been identified in all CD patients. Because of this, it is strongly suggested that a CD patient's immediate family (parents, sibling, and children) should be tested for CD. Statistics show that the immediate family members are also more prone to other autoimmune diseases. Aunts, uncles, cousins, and grandparents are also at risk, but to a lesser extent. The latest statistics indicate that when an individual with CD is diagnosed, another person in the immediate family has a 1 in 20 chance of having it also.

Further Research

Several other complications to CD have been mentioned in recent literature. Due to the fact that the prevalence of CD is increasing, the number of identified complications associated with CD is also increasing.

The quantity of research into CD and its complications is encouraging, in that eventually a vaccine, a medication, a genetically altered wheat with no gluten, or even perhaps a simple cure could be developed. But, until then, the best thing that a CD patient can do is to eat gluten-free.

CHAPTER 6

Tackling the Emotional Side of CD

Happiness comes of the capacity to feel deeply, to enjoy simply, to think freely, to risk life, to be needed.

—Storm Jameson

Celiac disease (CD) is one of the medical mysteries of this century. The obscure symptoms are like a complicated jigsaw puzzle . Only the frame of the puzzle is completed for now but, as research progresses, the complete picture will be seen. The mystery of CD will be solved, and the puzzle completed when all the at-risk groups are diagnosed.

Only another person with CD can comprehend the emotional aspects of CD. Living year after year with a variety of unexplained ailments is extremely frustrating. Those who experience the depression, anxiety, ataxia, or mental fogginess understand the significant impact this disease has on the individual and his family. It affects personal relationships, social situations, self esteem, and confidence. The majority of people with CD have been told, "It's all in your head." Family members many times may have developed the habit of "tuning out" their CD family member when they complain.

Eric Cassell describes suffering as: "A state of severe distress caused by events which threaten the integrity of a person." It could easily be said that "suffering" occurs in all CD patients *and* their families.

Because many physicians are still not aware of the prevalence of CD, they are looking for other conditions such as irritable bowel syndrome, chronic fatigue syndrome, fibromyalgia, or Crohn's disease, just to mention a few. This only delays a clear diagnosis of CD and prolongs the suffering.

CD will be recognized as a significant health problem when the pieces of the puzzle are found and the full impact is assessed; some believe that millions of CD patients are undiagnosed. CD may well be the disease of the next decade.

Common Emotional Reactions

Most newly diagnosed CD patients are subject to:

- Anxiety
- Insecurity
- Isolation
- Fear of the unknown
- Lack of information

Newly diagnosed CD patients need patience and understanding as they educate themselves to a new way of eating. This also applies to the parents of newly diagnosed children, who may feel helpless trying to find the information they need to have a healthy child.

Support Groups

Because doctors may not have the time to educate each individual with CD about the totally new way of life that the disorder demands, celiac support groups know the importance of support among peers. One support group, the Gluten Free Gang of Central Ohio, uses their group to discuss all new research, recipes, and restaurants in the area and offer support to new CD patients as they enter this new way of life. Here's a transcript of a typical meeting of the Gluten-Free Gang:

"The doctors should address the extreme emotions we experience, but it is rare," Lisa told the group. "After I was diagnosed I was overwhelmed with feelings of guilt and deprivation," Lisa explained. "I felt guilty complaining because many people have a life-threatening illness, such as cancer or multiple sclerosis. I felt guilty because I spent more money on my gluten-free food. I felt deprived because I could not eat exactly what I wanted. Then my feelings jumped back to guilt because people in Third World countries are really deprived of food, not me. The deprived feeling continued for about a year. It was hard to watch everyone dig into my birthday cake, which I couldn't even taste. Then I felt guilty because I was behaving like a child. Restaurant eating was frustrating when I couldn't order what I really wanted," Lisa concluded. "Then I was back to deprivation."

"My wife accused me of turning into a controlling husband because I wanted to become involved in meal planning and what restaurants we went to," Dean said.

"Things have gotten easier for me since I went to an open Alcoholic Anonymous meeting with my friend," Betty Jean said. "My friend explained that he could not drink alcohol because he would end up dead or in jail. He said I would kill myself if I did not eat gluten-free. He showed a lot of empathy for my situation because he just had to stay away from alcohol and I had to watch every drop of food I put in my mouth."

"Do you suggest AA meetings?" a member of the group asked.

"No," Betty Jean said as she laughed, "however, I do think it is a good idea to write down the Serenity Prayer that is said at each AA meeting. Each of us can use it as we adapt to our new way of eating."

The Serenity Prayer

God grant me the serenity to accept the things I cannot change,
The courage to change the things I can,
And the wisdom to know the difference.

"I can use that prayer when I get exasperated repeatedly explaining the disease to friends and relatives," a new member said.

"Think of yourself as a teacher educating the general public," said Maryalice. "You are clearing the path for celiacs in the future."

"What do you do when you are invited to a friend's home for dinner?' the new member asked.

"You can still accept dinner invitations or go to a potluck, just bring your own food. Don't change your social life," Lisa emphasized.

Emotions common to CD patients as they struggle to adapt to a new way of eating include:

- Relief at finally finding out what was wrong.
- Grief over the loss of lifestyle and food.
- Fear of eating something that will make them sick.
- Frustration in finding the right medical help.
- Difficulty in finding appropriate food.
- Difficulty in reading and deciphering labels.
- Difficulty in understanding and overcoming all aspects of depression.

Lucia, a member of the Gluten-Free Gang support group, offers this list of experiences common to all newly diagnosed CD patients:

Looking at a restaurant menu for the first time when trying to order a gluten-free diet (GFD), feeling apprehensive because time is ticking away, silently shedding a few tears, and feeling as if the task is too big to handle.

Trying to decide on a snack or a packed lunch so not to be singled out as different.

Trying to convince family and friends that you cannot go off a GFD "just this once" and "yes, it will hurt me."

Trying to explain ingredients that indicate gluten in labeling.

Taking two or three additional hours to shop for the family, and that before the trip to the health food store.

Making a daily decision regarding gluten-free ingredients.

Individuals with CD must recognize that they have undertaken a new way of life. These complex feelings are the norm, not the exception, and fortunately, these feelings do not last forever. But because this disease is virtually unknown, you must continually explain it to family, friends, co-workers, teachers, doctors, servers at restaurants, grocers, and many others, almost on a daily basis. When you consider how many contacts are made every day, the challenges are evident.

"Don't think it is the end of the world," Mary, another group member said. "It could be worse. Years ago, people did not have support groups or health food stores that now carry numerous gluten-free products. For those celiacs who live in small communities, there are many Internet vendors who also sell gluten-free foods.

"We must remember to mentor newly diagnosed celiacs," Mary reminded the group. "I can remember coming to my first support group feeling alone, confused, and needing the help of others. I think one of the main shocks was when I realized how life would be different due to the diagnosis."

When the mother of a recently diagnosed child walked into the meeting, the consensus of opinion was to ask Barb to share her story. When children are diagnosed with CD the parents have to make the largest adjustment.

"It is interesting to reflect back over the past 2 years since Natalie was diagnosed," said Barb. "So many emotions come flooding back. In hindsight, I wish we had pushed the celiac testing faster. We are in a minority because Natalie was diagnosed in less than 7 weeks from the first major symptom, though she showed many of the classic symptoms from about 9 months on.

"Dan and I had it pinpointed at about 3 weeks into testing by reading the *Merck Manual*, at our local library, after an upper gastrointestinal series of tests. The numerous tests scared us to death.

"My husband and I reacted very differently after the diagnosis. He was relieved and moved on. I, on the other hand, began to grieve for Natalie. I am getting better, but still have my days.

"I am already a compulsive person and, boy, did her diagnosis set that into overdrive! Nothing like coming home after the diagnosis and gutting your kitchen.

"One time, I remember we were 9 months into our new lifestyle, and I was driving back from my first Celiac Conference at Children's Hospital. I just burst out into tears and had to pull over. I kept thinking, 'How am I going to make life somewhat "normal" for Natalie and our family? How am I ever going to learn all of this? It is so overwhelming.'

"I have since thrown out the word 'normal' from my vocabulary as much as possible, and my learning curve is beginning to bend a little.

"As parents, Dan and I have to protect Natalie while teaching her to protect herself from food. She has to learn how to live in a gluten world, and we struggle each day over how to teach her how to do it.

"After our son was born, a dear friend told me, 'Parenthood is a lifetime of joy and worry.' Boy, has that phrase taken on even more meaning now. When we have bad days, we always say, 'This could be a whole lot worse.' And we know that it could. We thank God for what we have.

"We are all healthier because of Natalie and we know it.

"The Gluten Free Gang has been a blessing. Those of us with kids often struggle, since we are outnumbered by the adults. I have really focused on gathering up parents of children with celiac disease. Several are now coming back to the support group meetings.

"I also have tried to keep us all in contact via e-mail. With young families, it is hard to get to meetings, so we write each other as often as possible with questions, concerns, or just funny stories," Barb concluded.

Support and Education

Everyone at the meeting gave her a round of applause because, even though they might not have a child with CD, they were able to take courage, hope, and strength from her experience.

Living gluten-free is a choice for health's sake. When the alternative makes you a high risk for several forms of cancer, plus other catastrophic symptoms, it is understandable that each day you must make a deliberate decision to maintain a gluten-free life. This daily decision takes personal determination, family support, and a physician who is aware of how to treat CD.

The CD community offers an extended helping hand to new CD patients and to anyone who needs guidance in dealing with the disease. Physician's information is available through the CD community, to provide patient education and resource materials so that appropriate referrals can be made.

Many people with chronic diseases choose to go into a state of denial. This situation creates a condition in which the family must either "play act" to enable the denial or become confrontational and attempt to expose the denial. In this situation, an integrated health care team can identify the problem "up front."

CHAPTER 7

Raising a CD Child

You give them your love, but not your thoughts,
For they have their own thoughts,
You may house their bodies but not their souls,
For their souls dwell in the house of tomorrow, which you cannot visit, not even in your dreams.
You may strive to be like them but seek not to make them like you.
For life goes not backward nor tarries with yesterday.
You are the bows from which your children as living arrows are sent forth.

—Kahlil Gibran

Infants with celiac disease (CD) will usually show symptoms when grains (wheat, barley, or rye) are introduced into their diet. These symptoms will include diarrhea, foul-smelling stools, abdominal bloating, and probably abdominal pain. The appetite declines because of the symptoms. A noticeable change in the normal growth pattern will occur. It is not unusual for a child with CD to be in the lower percentile of height for his age. The general appearance of the child is what usually frightens the parents, because the child looks and acts sick.

According to a Reuters Health Report from May, 2005, the best time to introduce gluten-containing foods to children who are at risk for CD is between 4 and 6 months of age. The research indicates that introducing gluten-containing foods after that can increase the risk of disease.

Beth, a member of the Gluten Free Gang of Central Ohio support group, kept a journal on her daughter and shared her memories:

"When Allison was 6 months old, she was experiencing bouts of vomiting and diarrhea. I kept pressing our doctor to find out what was wrong, and he kept saying that it was the flu or it was related to her recent ear infections.

"She also stopped growing, and she lost weight from 6 months to 1 year old. After 6 months of frustration, I finally insisted the doctor check her out. He scheduled a series of upper gastrointestinal tests. He claimed nothing was wrong and recommended no further testing.

"I called Children's Hospital GI Specialist's office and scheduled an appointment. We had to wait 2 months, since I was not referred as an emergency by another physician.

"Since she was still very sick, I kept a list of all medications, each doctor's appointment, and a food diary. When we finally saw the specialist, it took half an hour just to communicate the data I had accumulated. He examined her and said that he wanted to run a few tests to rule out cystic fibrosis, but he was fairly confident that she had celiac disease.

"My husband reacted rather strongly when we got to the car. He felt the doctor was a 'quack.' Even when the tests came back positive, my husband did not agree with the gluten-free diet. When we finally agreed on the gluten-free diet, our daughter began to thrive and started gaining weight.

"She looks and acts healthy again, and we are very pleased with Dr. Bruce Crandall, who is a pediatric gastroenterologist at Children's Hospital in Columbus, Ohio."

This story conveys some of the problems that parents experience as they strive to get help for their child. Parents feel helpless when they know their child is sick, and their level of frustration heightens when they are told nothing is wrong or they have to wait months for an appointment. If a pediatrician is aware of CD, the next referral should be to a gastroenterologist. The specialist should immediately order antibody tests and an endoscopy.

During the diagnostic period, the child will continue to lose weight and maintain a certain level of irritability. And the parents are, of course, under stress while caring for a sick child and frustrated because they cannot kiss the hurt away.

The parents' protectiveness often turns into grief when they realize the kind of changes they must lead their child through. Parental emotions run a wide gamut as they learn about the disease: They feel helpless as they search for food their child can eat; they feel guilt when they realize they have made a mistake and caused their child pain; at times, their self-confidence drops to zero. Every parent wants their child to enjoy a birthday cake or a snack after school with their friends. This is when intervention is desperately needed.

Parents must recognize the importance of educating themselves about a gluten-free diet (GFD), because their child's life actually depends on the food they place in her mouth. A complete understanding of CD is very important. Parents can not sneak "just a taste" of a donut or a muffin to their child. It is not enough to read this chapter if you want to understand CD; you must start at the beginning of the book and study the disease as if your child's life depends on it, because your child's life *does* depend on it.

A positive attitude toward CD is extremely important because this is a lifelong diet. Support groups that contain other parents of CD children can offer help, including:

- Education, including books and literature
- Recipe sharing
- Lists of stores to shop for gluten-free foods

- Tips for snacks
- Emotional and social support
- E-mail communications and website research information

Education, a GFD, and emotional adjustment are all imperative for a CD child to live a good, healthy life. The importance of a support group cannot be emphasized enough. Knowing that others are going through the same thing takes away the feeling of isolation. The Internet support groups are also essential, and can help you assimilate the knowledge curve more quickly when utilized.

Children usually have the classic type of CD, and parents can see similarities when they share experiences with other parents. A parent must immediately start building the child's self esteem, even if they are still feeling overwhelmed and inadequate. This is when parents desperately need a support group.

Schools

Parents must encourage independence in the child's choices of food from an early age. When the child is in the first grade, he should be able to tell the class, "No, this is what I can eat, thank you anyway." Otherwise, he will always feel different and not have any control over his choices.

Schools must be made aware of CD children's needs. Educate the teacher and the class on CD. Make the teacher aware of what gluten is and what foods are allowed. Ask for a teacher/parent meeting to educate teachers, the school nurse, and the principal. Take printed material; having the printed word at their fingertips will make for fewer mistakes. Make a list for family and friends of common products that are acceptable. Offer to provide gluten-free snacks so that the other children can experience what your child does.

A positive environment will go a long way to allowing your child to be happy, healthy, and well adjusted. Teach him to realize that following a GFD will keep him healthy, prevent other diseases, and provide independence that many other children do not have.

Snacks

When your child is invited to bring snacks, many alternatives are available. Fruit bars, gluten-free cookies, individual fruit cups, and many commercial products are available. Each child with CD should carry a short explanation of the disease and the importance of eating gluten-free.

Always have a gluten-free snack handy in case one is not available. It is essential that your child feels responsible for what he eats. He must feel confident and self-assured in his decisions. Help him realize that "eating gluten-free" is a way of life.

CHAPTER 8

Eating and Baking Gluten-Free

Most of the shadows of this life are caused by standing in one's own shadow.

—Ralph Waldo Emerson

The transition to a gluten-free kitchen can be an exciting adventure, if change and choice are approached with the right mental attitudes. Each person decides from minute to minute, from hour to hour, and from day to day, exactly how to behave in a given situation. Each person makes the decision to either act or react. A reaction means we give the emotions permission to run the gamut. It can easily lead down a trail of anger, despair, agitation, and hopelessness. However, an individual can decide to be in control, to act and not react. Decide to pause and think about how it will feel to live a symptom-free life; picture the person you want to become, and then start acting like that person.

Make the decision to go down the happy road to a new gluten-free life. Instead of becoming overwhelmed, let's together find a safe haven in a gluten-free kitchen.

The kitchen is a safe haven for family and friends to talk, to share, and to eat. A person with celiac disease (CD) has the right to have a safe kitchen; however, it takes the cooperation of the total household to help make the kitchen a safe haven for a person with CD.

Celebrate the new transition with dignity. Set a table with special gluten-free snacks and light a candle. The light signifies the enlightenment brought into a person's life when CD is finally diagnosed. A light is needed to read and to gain knowledge. A light leads to understanding and consequently good health. It is fulfilling to enter the gluten-free diet (GFD) with ceremony and gusto.

The CD Safe Zone

Now, let's get to work. The right attitude is important as you prepare your kitchen. This is the beginning of living a symptom free life.

If you live alone, no problem. Simply remove all items containing gluten from the kitchen and start from scratch. Thoroughly clean each shelf, including each crevice and corner, to help assure that you live a symptom-free life. This method is not realistic if other people live in the house with you, because you must consider their needs as well.

Decide, with other members of your family, the exact area for the gluten-free shelves and counter space. Several shelves and an area of the counter should be considered your "safe zone."

This special area is important, because if a member of the family makes a wheat bread sandwich in the safe zone, and a few wheat particles from the bread contaminate food prepared for you in the same area, you could get sick. Make a sign to remind others that this is the "Celiac's Safe Zone."

Take the time to communicate with children. Make sure they understand the disease and what happens if food is contaminated with gluten. Children can help adults to obey the rules in a CD-safe kitchen.

All gluten-free products, whether in jars, bottles, cellophane, plastic, paper, cardboard, or Styrofoam, should be marked with a colorful sticker or marker, without exception. Some people prefer to purchase matching storage containers. This method can be very expensive; however, a trip to the dollar store can drastically reduce the price.

No one should touch gluten-free products without being overseen by you, the CD patient, or the person in charge of the kitchen. If a family member decides to borrow from the gluten-free supply while making a gluten-containing meal, they could contaminate the gluten-free container with gluten. Continue to explain, without hesitation, the importance of others following the kitchen rules so you can live without symptoms.

Have a special place in the refrigerator to keep food and leftovers. Separate bottles of mayonnaise, relish, mustard, and all other condiments should be marked with a sticker or a marker. Squeeze bottles work for the entire family because knives or spoons are not placed inside the container and the top can be washed.

Porous pans, cutting boards, stones, or wooden bowls or wooden spoons should never be used in the gluten-free area of the kitchen. Never use a food container if the interior surface cannot be scoured spotless.

Stainless steel pans, skillets, bowls, and utensils can be used in both areas of the kitchen, if a dishwasher is used between uses. Stainless steel containers can be used to prepare gluten-free food, and then rinsed out to prepare food for individuals on a regular diet. Remember, it is important to never use stainless steel containers for a GFD without going through the dishwasher first. The whole household can use trays as food preparation surfaces, as along as the trays are washed in the dishwasher after each use. An excellent place to purchase stainless steel items for the kitchen is at a restaurant supply store.

The gluten-free area should include its own pasta server and colander to use with gluten-free pasta.

Since it is not feasible to wash a can opener in the dishwasher after each use, you should have a special can opener. Examine the cutting edge of any can opener and traces of food can usually be found. If you think it's clean, just use a toothbrush in some of the crevices—it is easy to see why you need your own can opener!

Keeping the workspace continuously clean is essential. Pouring cereal out of a box close to the CD work area or clean dishes can cause contamination. Family members should be asked to use the sink when pouring items from a package into a cup or bowl. This habit helps to keep any spillage contained in the sink. By simply running water, the mess can be cleaned up.

> A single dad met on the Celiac chat line insisted that his three children use the sink when pouring cereal from the package to the bowl. They were also taught to open all boxes in the sink, including crackers and cookies. He trained them to use a cutting board over the sink when mixing or cutting items for a recipe. He was very proud to share his story, because this habit helped to keep the kitchen much cleaner than he thought possible.

Always place gluten-free items to be warmed in the microwave on a plate, so that they never touch the oven shelf. You seldom see a microwave without a crumb. It is important to cover food with a paper towel, paper plate, wax paper, or plastic wrap to prevent food that is adhered to the walls of the microwave from contaminating the gluten-free food.

A toaster oven has proven to be indispensable to many people with CD . The texture of gluten-free bread makes it difficult to toast in a regular toaster; besides, family members commonly use a regular toaster for wheat toast.

Toaster ovens come with various options and further help you to have another safe zone. When on a GFD, any option you can find will help to widen your food horizons.

Shirley, a lady in her fifties, called me panic stricken because she was diagnosed with CD. Her life revolved around food: every Wednesday, her Bridge Club met at a different house for lunch and an afternoon of Bridge; every Sunday her family gathered at a different house each week for fellowship and to see who could come up with the most delicious and unique dishes. Every Monday was spent with the "Restaurant Rovers," a group of people who went to different restaurants to eat. She spoke about her concerns and confessed she had not visited with her friends or family while she converted her kitchen and was learning how to cook gluten-free.

She had been quite verbal about her dislike of people complaining about physical symptoms. No one was aware she had any physical problems, and now she had to eat crow. She didn't want to explain CD to each individual member of her family, Bridge Club, and "Restaurant Rovers."

As we spoke, it was obvious she had a spacious home and enjoyed entertaining. I actually said very little as she talked through her concerns and came to a conclusion. She decided to invite everyone to her home for an evening of CD education. She asked me to speak. After I said yes, she asked me for an outline of my talk, because she wanted to hand out a brochure about CD.

I must confess, it was an evening I will never forget.

After everyone was seated at the tables, she tapped her sterling silver spoon on the crystal.

"Thank you for coming," she repeated several times until everyone gave her undivided attention. "We are here to celebrate the fact I have been diagnosed with celiac disease. We are not celebrating the fact that I have CD, but we are celebrating the fact that there is a solution. CD can remain in remission as long as I do not eat gluten. I thank God because

I have a disease with a solution," Shirley said, as she raised her wineglass and tilted her head toward the ceiling.

"I would like to introduce Sylvia Bower, a registered nurse and an individual living with CD. She will speak to us, after we eat, as we sip on our coffee. Please look at the CD brochure, lying by your plate, during the meal. It is very possible I am not the only person in this room with CD. Ms. Bower has also volunteered to stay and answer individual questions."

She served a multi-course Italian meal, starting with bruschetta on sesame rice crackers, followed by an Italian salad. The main course was a breaded veal cutlet, baked potato with sour cream and chives, and green beans almondine. Dessert was a wonderful crème brulle. She also served a delicious crusty, Italian bread (gluten-free).

Her friends were impressed with her originality. The food was delicious and, in addition to having a good time, everyone left with a clear understanding of CD.

The dinner's magnificent flavors surprised everyone. They were surprised the gluten-free flour mix, used to brown the veal cutlets, did not interfere with the flavor of the meat.

"I thank you for indulging me this evening," Shirley said to the group after the speaker. "Please continue to invite me to all of the gatherings; however, do not be offended when I pull out my little brown bag lunch made in my gluten-free kitchen. Please understand, as I want to be part of the solution to this disease by sticking to my gluten-free diet."

"Hey Shirley," her cousin yelled, "What are you going to do when we go on our retreat and have our big pancake breakfasts?"

"I get to use the skillet for my gluten-free pancake mix *before* you contaminate the skillet with your gluten pancakes," Shirley yelled back.

"Nothing is going to keep that gal down," said one diner.

The idea of cooking the gluten-free pancakes or other foods before putting gluten in the skillet also holds true for meat. Many homes only use gluten-free flour to brown meat and make gravies, because it decreases the chance of contamination and tastes quite good. The herbs and spices determine the taste more than the flour or batter.

Gluten Demystified

To learn how to cook gluten-free, it is necessary to understand gluten and just exactly what it does. Gluten is the protein substance in wheat, barley, and rye that holds the dough together and makes the flour pliable and thick and gives it the ability to be kneaded and to accept injected air. Gluten-free flour does not have any gluten to give it pliability. It is necessary to adjust recipes by adding xanthan gum and extra eggs to recipes to add the elasticity. The dough therefore becomes very thick, is sticky, and is not pliable.

Baking Gluten-Free

When you bake, you'll be using some ingredients you've probably never used before. A gluten-free cookbook should help in getting started on the new adventure of gluten-free cooking and baking, and many are out there on the market.

Bread is one of the most frequently missed items on a GFD. Making buns is an excellent way to solve that craving. There are many creative ways to individualize buns, such as adding onion flakes, poppy seeds, sesame seeds, herbs, cinnamon, and raisins. Muffin top tins or baking rings (English muffin rings) can be used. The muffin top tins allow for browning on the top and bottom. All bread and buns must be sliced as soon as they are baked and put into individual bags and frozen. This guarantees a fresh bun to satisfy the next craving for a sandwich. Buns can be made out of rice flour, potato starch, and tapioca flours, or by using a bean flour mix. The bean mix is more nutritious and contains more fiber, which is important because nutrition and fiber is sometimes lacking in some CD diets.

Each gluten-free kitchen should have on hand the following ingredients to make cooking and baking easier:

- Xanthan gum, gelatin, and eggs are used to hold dough together in all gluten-free baking.
- Rice flour (brown and white), if used alone, will be slightly gritty and anything made from it will fall apart easily. It works best if mixed with potato starch and tapioca starch. A combination of flours used in gluten-free recipes is available from Asian food stores (with a possible chance of contamination), health food stores, and on the Internet.
- Sweet rice flour, also known as gluten rice flour, is often called for in pastries or cookie recipes. It is a light, sweet flour and is available from Asian and health food stores.
- Bean flours are good if mixed with other types of flour. The most common are garfava (a mixture of garbanzo and fava beans), black bean, and mung bean flours. These are often mixed with sorghum flour, cornstarch, and tapioca starch. This flour is high in protein and fiber. It is available in some grocery stores and in health food stores.
- Soy flour is a heavy flour with a strong flavor. It can be used in small amounts but not as the main flour ingredient.
- Cornmeal and cornstarch are ingredients often used in gluten-free recipes. Cornstarch is commonly used for gravies and thickenings.
- Clear gelatin adds substance to gluten-free recipes. It is available in any grocery store or health food store.

- Rice bran, rice polish, arrowroot, nut flours, quinoa, buckwheat, and amaranth are also used in some gluten-free baking recipes.

All the above ingredients will be found in some of the commercially prepared gluten-free foods.

Breads

Gluten-free breads can be purchased from health food stores or through many Internet sites. Many varieties are available, both on the shelves and in the freezer. Gluten-free bread can be made at home either in a heavy-duty breadmaker or with a heavy-duty mixer and then baked in the oven. (A light-duty mixer motor will burn out from the heavy mixing required.) When making bread, cut it when it is cool and place each slice in a plastic bag and freeze. When ready to use, remove from the freezer and either thaw naturally or toast. If you are using a bread maker, it should be programmable so that there is only one mix and one rise. Red Star Yeast is very helpful in providing information and recipes for gluten-free bread.

Buns

A bread recipe is great for sandwich buns. To enrich them, try to find a recipe that uses bean flours, sorghum, or a combination with cornstarch and or tapioca starch. They will hold together better as a sandwich. This dough can also be used for bread sticks, cinnamon rolls, and pizza crust. The dough is sticky, because it does not have the gluten to make it pliable and stretchy.

Cakes

Many wonderful gluten-free cake recipes are available. After a while, it will be possible to adapt regular recipes to gluten-free ones. Adding xanthan gum is essential for all gluten-free baking. Cakes with nuts, raisins, carrots, and other dried fruit are moister and stay together better. Cheesecake is easy to adapt to be gluten-free, as are many other recipes. Cake mixes also can be purchased that are gluten-free. These are very good, especially when you are in a hurry.

Cookies

Gluten-free cookies can be purchased off the shelf at many grocery stores and health food stores, and from many Internet websites. Many recipes are available for home-made gluten-free cookies, too. Always use xanthan gum and never use a baking stone previously used with gluten dough.

> Gravies and Thickeners. Use rice flour, potato starch, corn starch, tapioca starch or a combination to make Hollandaise sauce, cheese sauce, or thickening for soups.

Summary

Remember to keep a good attitude and decide to act—not react—to your new way of life. Make your kitchen a safe haven where you can enjoy your family and friends and know you will not get sick from contaminated food. Be careful not to make the gluten-free kitchen a stressful experience. Words of encouragement to your family, including a thank-you for their cooperation, go much further than complaining. Do not hesitate to celebrate with that same candle that first brought the light leading to knowledge.

Enjoy a trip to the health food store and the Asian grocery story. Get a supply of prepared items. Some people will not want the full kitchen experience, but be sure to allocate a lot of time to reading labels. You might be surprised how much you enjoy cooking. It really is a satisfying experience to make a recipe with your own hands and then to receive immediate gratification by filling the stomach.

CHAPTER 9

Eating Out

To be without some of the things you want is an indispensable part of happiness.

—Bertrand Russell

The gluten-free diet (GFD) is "doable" at home; however, it is nice to eat out, at least once in a while. The first time you go to a restaurant as a celiac disease (CD) patient, you might think you are prepared, but when actually confronted with the situation, you might find yourself overwhelmed.

Restaurant Dining

When a group of people with CD discussed their first adventure eating out after being diagnosed, they found some common denominators: an overwhelmed feeling when looking at the menu and not knowing how to explain your special needs headed the list.

To simplify things, you might try handing your server the following card:

I have celiac disease. To avoid intestinal damage, I cannot eat any food product, chemical additive, or stabilizer containing even a trace of WHEAT, RYE, BARLEY, OATS, OR ANY DERIVATIVE OF THESE GRAINS.

Some common sources of these ingredients include: flours, thickeners, cereals, coating mixes, sauces, soy sauce, marinades, tenderizers, malt, malt flavoring, malt vinegar, modified food starch, pasta, croutons, stuffing, seasonings, self-basted poultry, imitation seafood, beer, broth, roux, and soup bases. If my food is cooked in a vat of oil or other cooking surface used for the above ingredients, it will be contaminated with gluten. Please use nonporous cookware or place aluminum foil on the grill before grilling my food.

I become ill if I eat any of the above foods.

Please check with the chef to make sure my food does not contain any of these ingredients.

I am able to eat foods containing cheese, milk, corn, potatoes, rice, fresh meat, poultry, or fish, fresh fruits and vegetables, garlic, olive and canola oil, butter, pure spice's and fresh herbs as long as they are prepared with none of the above ingredients.

Thank You Very Much

Most restaurants will try to accommodate your needs, once they understand them. A hand-out card makes the process much quicker and, if you're shy about asking for special foods, much easier, too.

Keep in mind that, when dining out, there is a difference between a "cook" and a "chef." Restaurants that employ cooks hire them to prepare food according to the dictates of a corporate office, owner, or manager. A cook follows orders and is not always aware of all the ingredients in certain dishes. A chef, on the other hand, has been trained in the culinary arts and is usually aware of special-needs diets, such as those prepared for diabetic and CD patients. She is a professional who wants to create a meal according to the individual diner's needs and tastes. In fine dining restaurants, your chef may come to your table, discuss solutions, and make recommendations. Once you understand the difference between a cook and a chef, you can determine how to approach each dining-out situation. It takes time to feel comfortable, but soon you will develop your own way of handling the situation.

It takes confidence to speak out about what you need and what will happen if you do not get it. Don't get sick just because your are too shy to speak out or because you do not want to call attention to yourself. Be polite, but be assertive. Being diagnosed with CD is a great time for a shy person to visualize the person she wants to become and then start acting like that person.

You're best bet is to find a locally owned restaurant where the servers are trained to cater to each customer's needs. If your server does not know the contents of menu ingredients,

Some national restaurants now offer gluten-free menus:

- Outback Steakhouse
- Bonefish Grill
- PF Chang's
- First Watch
- Wendy's
- McDonald's
- Don Pablos
- Carrabba's
- Chick-Fil-A
- Subway

Donato's Pizza has a No-Carb pizza with a gluten-free soy crust. Be aware, however, that many restaurants choose to be "legally" safe and not commit to serving gluten-free foods. These restaurants are concerned about becoming legally liable if a person with CD becomes ill through eating gluten-contaminated food.

ask to speak to the chef, briefly explain CD, show the chef your hand-out card, and ask for help in making a selection. Once you know you are being protected from gluten, you can relax and enjoy your meal. This type of restaurant may cost more, but the extra money is worth the peace of mind. It's not hard to understand why some restaurants refuse to commit to serving gluten-free meals. As more research is done on CD and on the gluten content of foods, knowing for certain what foods are and are not gluten free presents a moving target. For example, one CD organization maintains that white vinegar is not gluten-free, even though research has proven that the proteins of grains used to produce the vinegar do not survive the distillation process. The ingredients in many prepared foods may change over time, and just because something is gluten-free this year, it doesn't mean it will continue to always be gluten-free; you eat a familiar "safe" product and, because an ingredient was changed, you may become ill. It is your responsibility to determine what is gluten-free. Read labels. Ask questions.

The American Dietetic Association has been proactive in starting a group within their organization to identify and present the parameters of a gluten-free diet.

When reading a menu in a restaurant, look it over and decide what you want and how it will fit into the GFD. First rule out pasta, breads, breading, fried foods, croutons, flour tortillas, pita, or any other obvious item with gluten. Then decide on an entrée. Do not choose baked meat, fish, or fowl without checking with the cook or chef first, because sometimes special seasonings are rubbed on the outside before baking. Injections of special seasonings and tenderizers are occasionally used to enhance the flavor and tenderness of beef or pork roasts and sometimes chickens and turkeys. Bread stuffing is also commonly baked with meat, poultry, or fish. Broiled beef, pork, fish, or chicken is always safe if the only seasoning used is butter, garlic, salt, and pepper.

Next choose your side dishes. A baked white or sweet potato is always a good, safe selection. If in the mood for french fries, always check to make sure nothing else is cooked in the same oil. Oil used to prepare breaded onion rings, chicken, fish, or other breaded items will contaminate the oil with gluten and any food cooked in it.

Now choose your salad. Always specify "no croutons." Vinegar and oil dressing is always safe, except for malt vinegar made from barley. If another type of dressing is used, always ask to see the container so you can read the ingredients label or, if the dressing is made "in house," ask for the ingredients. (Many a server has had to carry a 2-gallon jar of salad dressing to the table for me to check the ingredients!) Most Italian and Ranch Dressings are gluten-free, but it is always wise to check. Most servers really do not mind providing this extra service, because they do not want their customers to get sick. Just remember, the more you can help to educate the public about CD, the sooner gluten-free food will be served without questions.

Probably the best example of what can happen when dining out occurred on my own birthday recently. My husband wanted to take me to a "nice" restaurant, so made reservations for a restaurant that was one of a chain of restaurants employing fully knowledgeable chefs and servers. The server came to take our order, and I explained my dietary needs. Since it was an Italian restaurant, he suggested that I order whatever dish looked good and then substitute the pasta for "something else." I ordered Gnocchi Vegetale, which was potato gnocchi with artichokes, roasted red peppers, broccoli, and mushrooms. I requested that shrimp be added instead of the gnocchi. He agreed that was fine. He checked with the chef a few times before we finally agreed. They served our salads, which were gluten-free. When the entrées came, mine had gnocchi pasta on the plate. The server took it away and apologized.

About 5 minutes later, he brought me a plate with shrimp and most of the above mentioned vegetables. When I was three-quarters of the way finished, I pulled a long egg noodle from my plate. When the server came to clear the plate, I explained that it had contaminated my food. The server again apologized. The manager credited us for my meal, and gave me a free dessert which consisted of blueberry sorbet, vanilla ice cream, and meringue. It was delicious. I completed a comment card about the incident and offered to teach the kitchen staff about CD.

About 3 hours later, I became very nauseated and had abdominal pain. Of course, the first thing that you think of is "is this my imagination or was my food really contaminated?" Well, usually when I suspect that I have had gluten, I take a dose of psyllium (Metamucil) in water to move the gluten through my system. I did that, but still had symptoms until about 2 A.M.

The moral of this story is that, no matter how long you are gluten-free and no matter how hard you try to control it, you are still at risk of eating gluten when dining out. It's important to educate others about CD.

> One of the advantages of being in a CD support group is hearing about places where it's safe to eat. Sharing these experiences, new recipes, and places to shop, makes the gluten-free lifestyle a little easier.

Remember, it is much easier on everyone if you identify your dietary needs to the server *before* the meal is served. If the steak comes served on a piece of bread, and you said nothing about specific needs, then it is your error, not the restaurant's. It is extremely important to emphasize to the server that no wheat, barley, or rye can be used in your meal.

I've found that going to Wendy's for a taco salad, or a chili and baked potato are always a "quick fix" when I get the urge to eat out. And an omelet is always safe—after your gut heals, you can even add the cheese.

> The recent low-carb diet craze has really helped those of us on a GFD. Restaurants no longer look with awe when you ask for "no bun."

When traveling, plan ahead for meals, taking into consideration how long the trip is and what will be available at the destination. Purchase gluten-free bread, crackers, cereal, snacks, and fruit. Pack a cooler so that an alternative is always available to fall back on.

When dining out with a CD child, always take along her favorite finger foods, so she'll be sure to get something she likes when they start eating out. Even though most children's menus include many gluten-filled items, most restaurants will cooperate so that the child can eat safely, gluten-free. Always encourage your child to try new foods; this helps them acquire tastes for a larger variety of foods. (For more tips on diets for CD children, see Chapter 6, "Raising a CD Child.")

Dining with Friends and Family

Friends and family can cause problems because they might not realize the dangers to you of not adhering to a GFD. You are sure to hear at least once, "Oh, that little bit won't hurt you, will it?"

Your response should be "Just as a diabetic cannot eat sugar, I cannot eat gluten because the consequences might be deadly."

It's a reply that might catch the attention of a family member or friend who has failed to understand the importance of your GFD. If the individual still makes no effort to understand CD and acquiesce to your needs, then it is very important to not give in. Remain firm and continue to take care of yourself, even if it means not eating what is being served.

Always take food with you when leaving the house, to eliminate the possibility of going hungry. Never hesitate to bring out your stash of gluten-free food when others are eating things you can't eat. It is important for you to continue to enjoy all your usual activities. Just remember that the reason for any activity is to gather together for a common cause and not just to eat.

If you are attending a banquet requiring advanced reservations, simply respond on the R.S.V.P. that a GFD is required, and most large banquet facilities will comply. In a small town or less-populated area, it may be necessary to take your own food. (On one such occasion, everyone else had to eat a pasta salad with dry stuffed chicken, while I was served a beautiful plate of roast beef and fruit. Being on a GFD sometimes has its perks!) Remember, it is the occasion that you are participating in, not just the meal. Don't let CD interfere with your social life.

After becoming comfortable with a GFD, sit down and make a list of the most common brand-name foods that are gluten-free. Copy this list and give it to your family and friends. Update the list yearly. They will appreciate your effort, knowing that they can take your needs into consideration when they are hosting a gathering. (They also will appreciate how many labels you need to read!)

A few organizations publish a shopping list that is updated annually. These organizations can be found in the Chapter 10 "Resources."

CHAPTER 10

Managing Celiac Disease

It is not what he has, nor even what he does, which directly expresses the worth of a man, but what he is.

—Henri Frederic Amiel

The National Institute of Health (NIH) Consensus Development Conference Statement on Celiac Disease, which was released on August 9, 2004 gives some excellent guidelines for managing the disease. Some of this may sound repetitious, but this is information that will soon be distributed to physicians. (If your doctor is not aware of the latest in CD management, take this with you.)

Managing Celiac Disease

Treatment for celiac disease (CD) should begin only after a complete diagnostic evaluation including serology (blood antibody tests) and biopsy (of the small intestine).

The management of CD is a gluten-free diet (GFD) for life. A GFD is defined as one that excludes wheat, rye, and barley. These dietary grains contain the peptides or glutens known to cause celiac disease. Even small quantities of gluten may be harmful. Oats appear to be safe for use by most individuals with CD, but their practical inclusion in a GFD is limited by potential contamination with gluten during processing. The strict definition of a GFD remains controversial due to lack of an accurate method to detect gluten in food products and the lack of scientific evidence for what constitutes a safe amount of gluten ingestion.

The following are six key elements in the management of individuals affected by CD:

- **C** onsultation with a skilled dietitian
- **E** ducation about the disease
- **L** ifelong adherence to a gluten-free diet
- **I** dentification and treatment of nutritional deficiencies
- **A** ccess to an advocacy group
- **C** ontinuous long-term followup by a multidisciplinary team

Learning about CD and how to identify gluten-containing products is associated with improved self-management. Participation in an advocacy group (support group) is also an effective means of promoting adherence to a GFD and may provide emotional and social support.

Following initial diagnosis and treatment, individuals should return for periodic visits with the physician and dietitian to assess symptoms and dietary adherence and monitor for complications. In children, this includes evaluation of growth and development. During these visits, health care providers can reinforce the benefits of adhering to a strict GFD for life.

Repeat serological testing may be used to assess response to treatment but is unproven. These tests may take a prolonged time (up to 1 year) to normalize, especially in adults, and may not correlate with improved histology. Persistent elevated serological levels may suggest lack of adherence to a GFD or unintended gluten ingestion. Individuals who do not respond to a GFD require re-evaluation. No established approach exists to screen for complications of CD, including lymphoma and adenocarcinoma of the small bowel.

Because the above statement was issued by a panel of experts in the field of treating CD, this is the most current and comprehensive opinion on managing the disease. In addition to the management guidelines, the NIH panel made recommendations for future research and presented a summary that is not only patient-oriented but verified by those who care for people with CD and are involved in research.

Educating the Public

It is true that the individual with CD must be responsible for his health and his diet. But it's empowering to learn more about your condition and be able to educate others regarding a disease that they probably have not heard of before.

Research into CD has increased by more than 100% over the last 5 years, and for that we can all be thankful. At this stage, education is the essential element. As newly diagnosed CD patients, their physicians, and other health care professionals are provided with up-to-date information, a more united effort toward managing the disease can be undertaken.

At a recent CD support group meeting, Carolyn stated that she felt that "Celiac disease is an ongoing challenge because of all of the variables and constant changes in items containing gluten." She said that even the manufacturers do not always know the source of starches used in processing. She also added that, "Many restaurants do not want to commit to what is gluten-free."

At the same meeting, Laura said that she found it difficult to convince her family that it was a life-long diet.

Bob said, "My fear is that my daughter will get it."

Ramona added, "I keep forgetting to tell my doctor to write on my prescriptions 'gluten-free.'" She said that she suspected she was getting gluten in her diet and later found that it was in her daily vitamin pills. Read *every* label.

Managing the disease on a daily personal basis is the goal of all people with CD. Each day, you must make a conscious effort to stay gluten-free. The prerequisites for a gluten-free lifestyle include:

- Reading all labels and knowing what you are eating
- Keeping a "safe zone" in your kitchen for gluten-free preparation
- Determining that your physician is aware of the follow-up needs of CD, such as assessing symptoms and dietary adherence and monitoring for complications and growth and development in children
- Creating an individual emergency program that will provide gluten-free foods in a crisis situation
- Having a restaurant hand-out card ready when eating out, especially when traveling
- Continuously informing family and friends of changes in the GFD, so that they are comfortable preparing foods for you
- For parents of CD children, communicating with school teachers and playmates and their families to make food choices easier for your child
- Knowing area grocery stores and resources in the area and informing grocers of the need for the availability of gluten-free foods.

Future Progress in CD Awareness

As CD patients, we can all help increase public awareness of the disease by enlisting the involvement of restaurants and food manufacturer's to produce and market more gluten-free items.

Speaking with one voice, through a single representative organization. would help:

- Establish the definition of gluten
- Collaborate with the American Dietetic Association to design and adopt a universal GFD

- Encourage the American Celiac Disease Alliance to continue lobbying for labeling laws that would identify the wheat, barley, and rye proteins on labels. (Effective in 2006, eight major food allergens, including wheat, will be identified on all food labels in the United States, thanks to the efforts of the CD Task Force.)
- Standardize serologic tests and pathologic criteria for the diagnosis of CD
- Determine the amount of gluten from wheat, barley, and rye that will cause pathology (small intestine destruction) in a person with CD

> *Gluten-Free Living*[1] has a great article by Amy Ratner regarding the European Union and its proposed regulations regarding food labeling. "The regulations specifically include grains containing gluten and all products derived from them. This will apply to 15 European countries. They do have a controversy on 'wheat starch,' which many European celiacs ingest. A trade association of European cereal starch processors states that 50% of all processed food in Europe contains a starch derivative.
>
> They did not take into account the extensive refining that occurs in the productions of starch derivatives. They had less than 0.01% protein and 'significantly' less gluten content than the 200 parts per million set as the Codex Alimentarius standard for gluten-free foods."
>
> What occurs in Europe will have a significant impact on the United States because the prevalence for CD in Europe and the United States is the same. (In Italy, all children are screened by age 7.)

A great necessity exists for uniting all persons with CD in the United States into a community that works for the common good. If this book accomplishes nothing else, my goal will be achieved.

---

[1]Ratner, Amy, "On the Other Side of the Atlantic," *Gluten-Free Living* 2004; Vol. 9, No. 2.

CHAPTER 11

Pulling It All Together

If you have knowledge, let others light their candles at it.
—Thomas Fuller

Walking the gluten-free life presents challenges. A challenge is not necessarily bad; it can be good. The first challenge is to get free of the symptoms of celiac disease by following a proper diet, but this is only the beginning. The next challenge is the healing process.

As the intestine heals, the body is finally able to start repairing itself. Before you are diagnosed with celiac disease, gluten is preventing your small intestine from absorbing the vitamins and nutrients your body needs to function. Each celiac patient knows how important it is for all parts of the body to work together.

Yet the healing process includes more than the body. Integrative medicine includes all the issues that affect your health: family, activities, diet, medications, stress management, and exercise. Even behavior-modification exercises can help you change actions or habits that are hindering your health.

To maximize your future health and happiness, it is important that you make an effort to bring your body, mind, and spirit into harmony. It is important to get into the driver's seat and to go past the disease as an obstacle. This is an easy statement to make, but let's see what it involves.

Healing the Body

When a celiac accidentally ingests gluten, it will usually cause symptoms such as bloating, gas, pain, or mental fogginess, which may last for two to three days. Some celiacs do not have symptoms but are aware that they have ingested gluten. The first course of action in either case should be to take a psyllium-based fiber laxative immediately, which will help clear the intestinal tract.

Follow a healthy diet

Getting enough fiber on a regular basis (35 g daily) will assist you in maintaining a healthy body. It will prevent constipation and provide bulk for celiacs with diarrhea. Because of the permeability of the small intestine with this disease (also called "leaky gut"), food either moves too slowly (causing constipation) or too rapidly (causing diarrhea).

Gluten-free foods are usually high in fat and carbohydrates because foods that are processed to *reduce* fat or carbs are likely to have gluten in them (read the labels). Switching to gluten-free foods can result in weight gain, especially in the first few years. Simple statements can't be made about losing weight; however, stress is also a common denominator for both the underweight and overweight. Others suffer from the opposite problem: weight loss. Nutritional drinks, high in calories and nutrition, can be used between meals to help an individual gain weight. Ice cream is delicious mixed with some of these drinks and increases the calorie intake.

Terry, from the Gluten-Free Gang, states that weight gain or reduction has been an ongoing endeavor for her.

"I've been overweight most of my life, except when I was real sick with CD," Terry told the Gluten-free Gang. "As most of us do, I packed on the pounds after going gluten-free. It took a long time for me to figure out what I was doing wrong, so I've made a list of what was happening and why. Maybe I can help someone else not make the same mistakes." (See Table 11-1)

Table 11-1 Terry's List

(a) After I went on a gluten-free diet, I was feeling hunger pangs as early as 20 minutes after eating dinner. Not because I needed the calories, but because my body was playing catch-up with nutrients.

(b) Gluten-free products are usually higher in fat and overall calories. If one eats the same number of gluten-free cookies as regular cookies, a person will take in a lot more calories. When wheat flour is not used, the substituted "texture" contains more calories and fat.

(c) A lot of time, I was eating the whole box of gluten-free cookies because "I could." Once I found a good-tasting product, I would go overboard and eat too much. Yes, this was definitely emotional eating; however, it was still necessary to deal with this issue as part of the bigger picture.

(d) Not that I want to make specific recommendations, but Weight Watchers has been successful for me. It is a flexible plan that accommodates my needs, and it really emphasizes healthy eating. There is no magic bullet to losing excess weight. Whatever method a person decides to use, it is always calories in versus calories out, healthy food choices to help the body heal, and activity to help the process along.

(e) I eat much less gluten-free bread and baked products than I did previously. This decision was not made because I cut my carbohydrates (carbs)—I need a lot of carbs because I ride a bike. I need my diet to include 60% to 75% healthy carb calories on the days I ride long distances. I choose more complex and unprocessed carbs that are gluten-free, such as breads, brown rice, pasta, quinoa, and buckwheat

Continued

Table 11-1 (Continued)

cereal. These items contain a good nutritional punch. Certainly, I eat cookies or cake on occasion, but I choose foods more often on the basis of quality over quantity.
(f) Fruit and vegetables are friends. One can have a lot of "friends" for not many calories.

Work with your doctor

When CD is diagnosed, the individual has to be preoccupied with the new gluten-free diet. Watching calorie intake is the farthest thing from one's mind; consequently, someone who had previously worked hard to *gain* weight may end up on a diet to *lose* weight. This problem is usually not expected; it creeps up insidiously.

It is important to follow up with your physician on a regular basis. The doctor will know by the symptoms if your intestine is healing and if your body is absorbing enough nutrition. All current symptoms will be evaluated, along with previous problems such as anemia, overweight, underweight, irregular heartbeat, diarrhea, or constipation. Continuous diarrhea may be an indication the individual is continuing to ingest gluten. Constipation forces the individual into a continuous awareness of fiber intake. On the other hand, a person with *dermatitis herpetiformis*, for example, may have lesions months after diagnosis even if on a gluten-free diet. Many celiacs have no more symptoms. Therefore, the symptoms found at the start of the disease determine the necessary follow-up.

Your physician will also consider the effects that CD has on your body and make a plan to evaluate them. For example, if you have not had a bone scan for osteoporosis, that should be done every few years until it is known whether damage has been done to the bones. Blood calcium, magnesium, folate, iron, vitamin B_{12}, and vitamin D may be monitored for absorption as proof of healing.

You need a physician who makes you feel empowered, since health is a state of well-being. Have a list of questions ready when visiting your physician. Continue to go over each question until each is answered to your satisfaction. Communication is very important, and if your questions are not answered, consider going to another physician.

Keep a diary

Whenever symptoms appear and you are not sure if they are celiac-related, start a two-week food diary to determine what is causing the symptoms. It may be a food allergy, a vitamin or medication containing gluten, or an item you normally eat, previously gluten-free, that may have new or changed ingredients.

SUNDAY	MONDAY	TUESDAY	WEDNESDAY	THURSDAY	FRIDAY	SATURDAY

Improve your lifestyle

In 1967, Frank Speizer began a Nurses Health Study with about 80,000 nurses participating. It was comprehensive and very successful because many of the nurses participated for at least 25 years. It started with an emphasis on women's health, but produced such comprehensive and useful results that a second study and a third study were done. The most important result of these studies was to reveal actual lifestyles that lower the risk of diseases. By controlling activities in our lives, eating or abstaining from certain foods, or realizing and compensating for our genetic risks, we can become healthier individuals.

Exercise is probably the most underestimated activity that benefits the whole body. The intestinal tract moves more easily, the muscles are toned, the cells are nourished, and the body can maintain a steady weight with daily exercise.

Exercising is taking care of the body. All exercises should start with stretching. When you start to age your muscles will degenerate if they are not used. Aerobic exercises help keep your body functioning by raising your heart rate to at least 120 beats per minute. The most recent suggestions state that 20 to 30 minutes per day of aerobic exercise is necessary for a healthy body. That could include walking at two to three miles an hour or walking on a treadmill.

After one has been sick, being depressed and feeling inadequate are not unusual for a period of time. When overcoming any type of illness the mind becomes sluggish. Taking care of the physical body can help our mental attitudes.

Healing the Mind

Realizing that the body is controlled by the mind is the first step to healing. The rigors of everyday life lead us to be so "busy" that we fail to take the time to just "be." Savoring life instead of just rushing through it results in a more balanced life.

Time each day must be allotted to pampering yourself. Soak in the tub or stand in the shower and permit the relaxing water to help relax your body. A shower chair can give many of the same benefits as a bath. Water removes germs, removes odors, and cleans the skin. Each day a person can walk into the water dirty and walk out clean. Taking the time to prepare your body for the day is a privilege.

Knowing you are clean from head to toe gives you a confidence not found any other way. A tap of powder in the shoes takes very little time. Keeping the fingernails and toenails cut, clean, and buffed helps to give the body that finished look.

Now is the time to start the diary. Make a daily note of exactly what you do to take care of your body inside and out. This notebook could include any physical symptoms you encounter and what you have to eat at each meal.

Have you ever noticed that helping and encouraging others gives you a sense of self-worth? Bernie Siegel in his book *Prescription for Living* states that encouragement is "the helium of life." Experiencing CD can be a challenge. We have the choice of making up our minds to:

1. Live gluten-free
2. Read all of those labels
3. Find a recipe that fits something that we really crave or feel deprived of
4. Find personal courage to not limit our social activities because of CD
5. Encourage other celiacs and feel better about ourselves
6. Have an attitude of gratitude
7. Develop a belief system that will provide you with confidence and hope

Become self-motivated. Determine what motivates you, look at what you value, and ask what is your purpose here in this life. Being thus empowered permits you to be confident and in control.

Thoughts have a definite effect on our body. When the body receives a message of despair, it sends signals through the central and autonomic nervous systems to *beware* that something is wrong. This can make our pulse rate rise and create panic attacks, anxiety, shortness of breath, and other physical symptoms. So how our mind reacts to things really does affect our physical health.

Healing the Spirit (Soul)

We are really three-in-one individuals because we do have a body, mind, and soul. It is impossible to separate them (Figure 11-1). It is much more effective if we allow them to work together.

Researchers have diligently studied the influence of the mind and spirit upon the body. Public television recently released a program with up-to-date information on this topic. The program, entitled *The New Medicine*, was hosted by Dana Reeves, who had terminal cancer at the time. It presented striking evidence about the direct effects of a person's state of mind on the healing process.

In celiac disease, an autoimmune disease, the body reacts to the individual's state of mind. There are many ways the immune system's functioning can be improved if we educate our mind and spirit. The antibodies in CD are

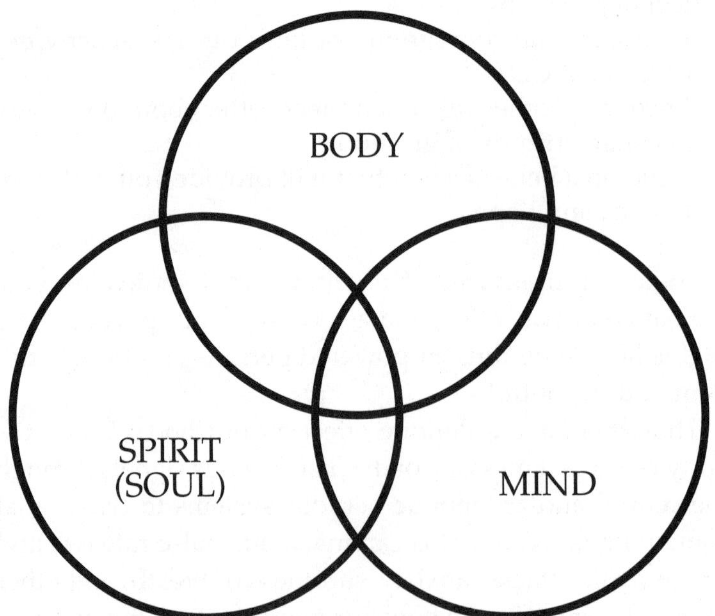

Figure 11-1. The intersection of body, mind, and soul (spirit).

reacting to the proteins penetrating our "gut" or small intestine. These proteins do not belong outside of the small intestine, so the body responds by producing T-cells. These T-cells can increase and allow lymphoma and other cancers to occur. The reason it is called *autoimmune disease* is that the body creates these antibodies against the proteins. Speaking simply, all autoimmune diseases are reactions to proteins that the body is trying to reject.

Dr. Bernie Siegel asks (in his book *Prescription For Living*) "What lifts your spirits and allows you to overcome difficulties? The answer is very simple: encouragement."

Set aside a quiet time each day to contemplate your goals and plan for the day. This is a good method for obtaining control over your mind. Keep a record of your mental attitudes and how you are working to improve them.

Each person decides on a minute-to-minute basis exactly what they will think, what they will say, and what they will do. Each of us must take full responsibility for our own behavior. The mind is like a computer and the owner of the brain is the programmer. If you are not satisfied with your attitudes, moods, temper, or words, you can change them. Write down in the notebook exactly how you want to change. Visualize the person you want to become and then start acting like the person you are becoming. Set time aside each day to do this visualization, along with a meditation.

Dealing with family members can sometimes be exasperating; however, it is extremely important, for our own peace of mind, to realize we cannot change anyone except ourselves. If you want to change another person, try changing yourself instead—make an effort to act and not react. It works.

Everyone should have a certain amount of time set aside to enjoy or explore hobbies or interests such as arts, sports, reading, fishing, or whatever gives their lives fulfillment. Family members are not going to tell a spouse, parent, sibling, or child, "Why don't you take some time off just for yourself?" It is important to sit down and explain to your family that this is part of the healing process. Taking time for yourself is not selfish; it's just common sense. It helps you live a balanced life.

You can use meditation, prayer, yoga, or visual imaging to center your thoughts on something meaningful. These techniques will reduce your stress and increase your capacity for hope.

How do we deal with adversity? Remember, if a tree is not pruned, it will not produce fruit. We are spirits; souls. Our bodies can be crushed, but faith and love continue to be a part of us. As celiacs, we are physically changed (by wheat damaging our small intestine), but our spirits and minds are still intact. That is why we need to know who we are as a person—so that when anything happens to our physical body, *we* remain the same. Remember, too, that it takes time to absorb major life changes.

The most difficult person that I have to deal with is me. I have to learn to be honest and love myself as the creature that God created before I can set my other priorities in life. If you put faith first in your life, then personal satisfaction will permit you to put your family and other relationships in order after that. That will lead to a life of service and creativity, which is why we were created: to be of service to each other. This gives equilibrium to the body, mind, and spirit.

Dr. Dale Matthews, in *The Faith Factor*, states that we "heal the body by restoring our physical selves" and we "heal the mind by finding a lasting peace."

There have been several studies done to evaluate the value of prayer, yoga, and meditation on healing. In *Prescription For Living*, Dr. Bernie Siegel cites the example of Dr. Alijani, a devout Muslim who found support in his medical practice in his faith. He believes that faith plays a significant role in his patients' well-being. "On the basis of my experience, the mind of the individual plays a major role in the healing process. What stands out above all is his or her faith. If you have faith, you will be a well-balanced, resilient person, prepared to solve the problem."

Many people believe that prayer is a literal lifeline. Research has indicated that prayer is effective, whether by the individual or intercessory prayer by others. This is irrespective of one's belief system. There are many examples in Eastern religions of individuals being able to walk on hot coals or beds of nails with no pain because of their ability to control their minds. Healing is a state of mind that needs to be nourished and cultivated. Hope is the central path of healing.

We have a multi-faceted body, and we are also multi-faceted beings. The total person is not just the body, not just the mind, and not just the spirit (or soul). A total person is body, mind, and spirit. All three must be integrated and work in harmony for you to attain your full potential.

CHAPTER 12

Gluten in Medications

by Steve Plogsted

Patients with celiac disease (CD) must be wary of gluten in pharmaceutical products. Gluten in pharmaceuticals is found in the inactive ingredients known as *excipients*. Excipients are pharmacologically inactive substances that are included the final formulation of the drug product. The purpose of the excipients is multifunctional. They provide bulk to the product, allow for the drug to be dissolved and absorbed at different rates in the body (as in extended release formulations), decrease stomach upset, protect the product from moisture contamination, and simply make the final drug appearance more pleasing to the eye of the consumer. The shape and overall appearance of the final product also helps in identification.

The U.S. Food and Drug Administration (FDA) has the authority to approve all drug products produced for legal use in the United States. Each drug product must undergo rigorous testing before it can be approved for marketing to the consumer. The proprietary or "brand name" drugs have to meet standards for dissolution, absorption, blood levels, product stability, and several other factors. The manufacturing facilities where the drugs are produced must maintain specific standards in regards to quality control, cleanliness, and packaging. The equipment used to manufacture the drugs undergoes extensive cleaning and maintenance to assure that none of the products are contaminated by unwanted matter. Closed-containment equipment should be used whenever feasible and when not, appropriate precautions are employed to prevent contamination. Workers are gowned, gloved, and masked to avoid human contamination and to protect the workers from the medication. Many of the pieces of equipment are dedicated to one product, but if a piece of equipment is used for more than one product, it is cleaned and sterilized or sanitized. Computers are employed extensively to ensure constant quality throughout the process. The manufacturers must maintain detailed records of every step of the process and are subject to constant surveillance by various government agencies.

The federal government also is involved in the content of the package insert that accompanies each drug product. The entire process can run into the hundreds of millions of dollars, which represents a sizeable investment for the drug manufactures. Generic drug manufacturers must adhere to the same standards but do not have to invest in the research to the same extent as do proprietary manufacturers. The products do have to demonstrate that their action is the same as that of the previously approved proprietary product. This means that the active ingredient(s) must produce the same pharmacologic response, but the manufacturers are free to produce a final product that differs in shape, color, texture, and excipients. These products are rated by the FDA as equivalent depending on whether the generic conforms to all the federal standards for that drug product. Those that do not conform cannot be legally substituted by the pharmacist but can be dispensed upon the physician's authorization.

Excipients added during manufacturing may be from a wheat source including unspecified starch, pregelatinized starch, dusting powder, flour, and gluten. Dextri-maltose and caramel coloring, which may contain barley malt, may be a source of gluten. Other starch derivatives such as sodium starch glycolate, dextrin, and maltodextrin are usually derived from potato starch or corn starch in North America, and so should be acceptable for CD patients, but caution should be used until the gluten-free status can be confirmed. Pharmacists and physicians may often be called upon to determine whether a pharmaceutical product is gluten free. This can be a challenging task. In a survey performed in 2001, only 5 of 100 pharmaceutical companies had a policy ensuring gluten-free status for their medications, although many more stated that they believed their products to be gluten free. One of the problems faced by the pharmaceutical manufacturers is the uncertainty of the gluten-free status of the raw materials obtained from outside sources. Cross-contamination during manufacturing of the excipients can also occur but is very unlikely in the manufacturing of the actual drug product.

A reliable way of determining the gluten-free status of the medications that they are taking is essential to the health of CD patients. Several books and websites are available to assist in this process, but should be thought of as starting places. If possible, inquiries should be made directly to the pharmaceutical companies to ensure the gluten-free status of a particular product. Adding to the burden of the CD patient is the fact that pharmaceutical manufacturers may change the inactive ingredients of their products. This can happen without warning, so the gluten-free status of a product should be re-assessed on a regular basis. Any indication that a product is "new and improved," "new formulation," "new product appearance," or "new manufacturer" should be a sign that the gluten-free status of the product must be re-established.

Table 12-1 is a short list of some of the common excipients ingredients used in the manufacturing of pharmaceutical products.

Table 12-1. Excipient Ingredients in Medications

Benzyl alcohol—Made synthetically from benzyl chloride, which is derived from toluene (a tar oil).

Cellulose (methylcellulose, hydroxymethylcellulose, microcrystalline, powdered)—Obtained from fibrous plant material (woody pulp or chemical cotton).

Cetyl alcohol—Derived from a fat source (spermaceti, which is a waxy substance from the head of the sperm whale).

Croscarmellose sodium—An internally cross-linked sodium carboxymethylcellulose for use as a disintegrant in pharmaceutical formulations. It contains no sugar or starch.

Dextrans—Sugar molecules.

Dextrates—Mix of sugars resulting from the controlled enzymatic hydrolysis of starch.

Dextrins—Result from the hydrolysis of starch (primarily corn or potato) by heat or hydrochloric acid. It can also be obtained from wheat, rice, or tapioca.

Dextri-maltose—A sugar that may be obtained from barley malt.

Dextrose—A sugar that is obtained from corn starch.

Fructose—A sugar also known as levulose or fruit sugar.

Gelatin—Obtained from the skin, white connective tissue, and bones of animals (by boiling skin, tendons, ligaments, bones, etc. with water).

Glycerin—Historically, glycerin (also known as glycerol), was made through:

* *Saponification* (a type of chemical process) of fats and oils in the manufacturing of soaps.
* *Hydrolysis* of fats and oils through pressure and superheated steam.
* *Fermentation* of beet sugar molasses in the presence of large amounts of sodium sulfite.

Today, it is made mostly from propylene (a petroleum product).

Continued

Table 12-1. (Continued)

Glycerols—Obtained from fats and oils as byproducts in the manufacture of soaps and fatty acids (may also be listed as mono-glycerides or di-glycerides).

Glycols—Products of ethylene oxide gas.

Iron oxide (rust)—Used as a coloring agent.

Kaolin—A clay-like substance.

Lactinol—Lactose derivative.

Lactose—Lactose, or milk sugar, is used in the pharmaceutical industry as a filler or binder for the manufacture of coated pills and tablets.

Maltodextrin—A starch hydrolysate that is usually obtained from corn but can also be extracted from wheat, potatoes, or rice.

Mannitol—Derived from monosaccharides (glucose and mannose).

Polysorbates—Chemically altered sorbitol (a sugar).

Povidone (crospovidone)—Synthetic polymers.

Pregelatinized starch—A starch that has been chemically or mechanically processed. The starch can come from corn, wheat, potatoes, or tapioca.

Shellac—A natural wax product used in tablet or capsule coating.

Sodium lauryl sulfate—Derivative of the fatty acids of coconut oil.

Sodium starch glycolate—A starch that is usually obtained from potatoes but may come from any starch source.

Stearates (calcium, magnesium)—Derived from stearic acid (a fat; occurs as a glyceride in tallow and other animal fats and oils, as well as some vegetables; prepared synthetically by hydrogenation of cottonseed and other vegetable oils).

Sucrose—Refined sugar also known as refined sugar, beet sugar, or cane sugar.

Titanium dioxide—Chemical used as a white pigment; not derived from any starch source.

Triacetin—Derivative of glycerin (acetylation of glycerol).

Silicon dioxide—Dispersing agent made from silicon.

CHAPTER 13

Gluten-Free Recipes

The Gluten-Free Gang Celiac Support Group in Columbus Ohio, participates along with Children's Hospital in an annual Celiac Conference. Each year a group of recipes is collected from celiacs which is then given to participants at the conference. When the Gluten-Free Gang was asked what should be included in this book, they all agreed that it should have recipes. After all, CD is a diet related disease and because there are restrictions, it is great to know some good things to prepare.

These recipes were submitted by our members as a courtesy to one another, and they include some of the group's favorite recipes. They are not meant to replace a cookbook, but offer ideas to the new celiac so that they may know that there are many options in preparing a meal.[1]

---

[1]These recipes were reprinted with the permission of the Gluten-Free Gang website (www.glutenfreegang.org).

Kitchen Basics

Darry's GF Flour Mix

(from Darry Faust, 2005 Conference Cookbook)

Ingredients:

3 cups	Rice flour
1 cup	Corn starch
3 cups	Tapioca flour
1/2 cup	Soy flour (optional)

Directions:

1. Blend in a large sturdy plastic bag and keep in the refrigerator for use as needed.

*****

GF Shake-n-Bake

(from Jodi Carlson, 2001 Conference Cookbook)

Ingredients:

2 cups	Dry GF bread crumbs
1/4 cup	Cornstarch
1 tbsp.	Paprika
2 tsp.	Salt
2 tsp.	Sugar
2 tsp.	Onion powder
3/4 tsp.	Oregano
3/4 tsp.	Garlic powder
1/4 tsp.	Cumin (optional)
1/4 cup	Vegetable shortening

Directions:

1. In food processor, whirl bread crumbs until fine.
2. Mix other dry ingredients and cut in shortening.
3. Store in covered container in cool, dry place.

*****

GF Fry Magic

(from Jodi Carlson, 2001 Conference Cookbook)

Ingredients:

1/2 cup	Cornstarch
1/2 cup	Potato starch
1/4 cup	Cornmeal
1/2 tsp.	Baking soda
1/2 tsp.	Xanthan gum
1 tsp.	Salt and pepper

Directions:

1. Toss all in plastic bag to mix.
2. Rinse meat to be fried and toss with coating mix.
3. Fry as usual.

*****

Thick Crust Pizza Dough

(from Darry Faust, 2005 Conference Cookbook)

Ingredients:

1 1/4 cup	Rice flour (white or brown)
1 cup	Tapioca flour
1/4 tsp	Xanthan gum
1 pkg	Unflavored gelatin
1 tsp	Baking powder
1 tbsp	Sugar
3/4 cup	Cottage cheese
1/8 cup	Olive oil
1/2 cup	Buttermilk
1	Egg, blended with fork

Directions:

1. Mix dry ingredients thoroughly.
2. Mix in wet ingredients.

3. This dough should be mixed and then formed into ball with a rubber spatula.
4. Dust the dough ball with rice flour. Roll out on rice flour dusted wax paper sheet.
5. Roll to about 1/2" thickness (or about 12" in diameter to fit a pizza pan).
6. The pizza can be cooked on a cookie sheet also. Flute the edges of the pizza shaped dough.
7. Bake 350 degrees for 30 minutes.
8. Spread sauce over the top of the pre-baked pizza dough. Top with your favorite toppings.
9. Bake 350 degrees for 10–15 minutes.

Tip: Slice and enjoy.

*****

BREAKFAST

Breakfast Brunch Casserole

(from Carolyn Randall, 1999 Conference Cookbook)

Ingredients:

6 cups	GF bread cubes or crumbs
1 1/2 cups	Cold milk
10	Large eggs, beaten to mix well
1 cup	Buttermilk
1 tsp	Dill weed
1 tsp	Mrs. Dash
4	Green onions, chopped
1 1/2 cups	Extra sharp cheddar cheese, shredded
1/2 cup	Finely chopped green or red sweet pepper
1 cup	Ham, chopped small
10 oz pkg	Frozen chopped spinach or chopped broccoli thawed and drained.

Directions:
Place the bread cubes or crumbs in a large bowl and heat in the microwave, stirring occasionally until bread is warmed through. Immediately pour the milk over the bread, stir well, and allow to stand. Coat a 9 x 13 glass baking dish with cooking spray. Put the eggs into a large container and mix well with a fork or whisk. Stir in the buttermilk, pepper, dill weed, and Mrs. Dash seasoning. Stir in the onion, green pepper, grated cheese, meat, and spinach or broccoli. Stir the egg mixture into the bread and milk, stirring to thoroughly blend. Pour this mixture into the baking dish.

It may be stored in the refrigerator, covered until ready to bake (next day). Preheat oven to 350 degrees and bake for one hour or until knife comes out clean.

*****

Corn Pancakes

(from Sylvia Bower)

Ingredients:

2 tbsp	GF flour
13-14 oz.	Cream-style corn
1 Tbl.	Vegetable oil
2	Eggs

Directions:
1. Combine all ingredients in a bowl.
2. Cook as you would any pancake on the griddle.

Optional: To "hide" corn, process in a blender in step one.

*****

Early Wake-Up Call

(from Pat Rudolph, 2005 Conference Cookbook)

Ingredients:

6	Eggs, beaten
1 lb	Monterey or mozzarella cheese, shredded
1 lb	Cottage cheese
1 cup	Milk
1 cup	GF Bisquick mix
1/4 lb	Margarine, melted
1 tsp	Parsley flakes
1 tsp	Dried onions
1 sm can	Chopped green chilies

Directions:

1. Blend together all ingredients and pour into 9 x 13 glass casserole.
2. Bake at 350 for 40 minutes or until toothpick comes out clean in the center.

Tip: You can use 1/2–3/4 lb cheese if using calcium fortified Lactaid Skim Milk, because this milk thickens well.

*****

English Muffins

(from Darry Faust, 2005 Conference Cookbook)

Ingredients:

1-1/4 cup	Rice flour
1 cup	Tapioca flour
1/4 cup	Powder milk
1 tsp	Xanthan gum
2 tsp	Baking powder
1 cup	Cottage cheese
3/4 cup	Water
2 tbsp	Olive oil

Directions:

1. Mix dry ingredients thoroughly.
2. Add wet ingredients and mix thoroughly.
3. Form a dough ball with the mixing spoon.
4. Dust with rice flour to make a cannon ball shape that rolls around the bowl without sticking.
5. Roll out the dough on a rice flour dusted length of wax paper.
6. Roll to 3/4-in. thickness. Cut out biscuits, any size. A 4-in. biscuit cutter will make about six biscuits.
7. Use spatula to lift off as the biscuits are cut. Re-roll the dough as needed to make the biscuits.
8. Place on cookie sheet. Parchment paper works very well.
9. Bake at 350 degrees for 30 minutes. No need to turn the biscuits over during baking.
10. Cool on a wire rack until thoroughly cool. Keep refrigerated.

Tip: These muffins taste great when toasted.

*****

Gluten-Free & Dairy-Free Pancakes

(from Heidi Hower, 2005 Conference Cookbook)

Ingredients:

1-1/4 cup	Bob's Red Mill All-Purpose GF Baking Flour
1 tbsp	Baking powder
1 tbsp	Sugar
1/2 tsp	Salt
1 tsp	Xanthan gum
1	Egg
1 cup	Milk or milk substitute
2 tbsp	Safflower oil

Directions:

1. Mix all ingredients in bowl just until blended.
2. Cook on hot griddle until golden brown on both sides.

*****

Sunday Morning Waffles or Pancakes

(from Darry Faust, 2005 Conference Cookbook)

Ingredients:

1 cup	GF flour mix*
1 tsp	Baking powder
3/4 tsp	Baking soda
1	Egg, blended
1 cup	Buttermilk
1 tbsp	Olive oil

Directions:

1. Mix dry ingredients thoroughly.
2. Mix wet ingredients thoroughly with spoon and let stand for about 5 minutes.
3. Ladle onto griddle: Pancakes will rise normally. Flip and cook both sides. Medium-low heat on an electric skillet works well.
4. Waffles: Normal cycle in preheated waffle maker.

**See Darry's GF Flour Mix on page XX*

*****

MAIN MEALS

Aunt Carol's Spinach Casserole

(from Jane Ehrenfeld, 2004 Conference Cookbook)

Ingredients:

10 oz. pkg	Spinach
1/2 cup	Mayonnaise, scant*

1	Egg
1/4 cup	Grated cheese (cheddar, parmesan, or other hard cheese)
1 tbsp	GF bread crumbs or cornflake crumbs (optional)

Directions:

1. Cook and drain spinach according to directions on package. (In microwave or on stovetop, it doesn't have to be very cooked beyond thawed enough to drain.)
2. Drain all excess liquid. (I use cheesecloth and squish by hand. The more you drain the better the dish turns out.)
3. Mix spinach with approximately 1/2 cup mayo, egg, and cheese. Can be done in the same dish as baking. Just wipe edges before putting in oven.
4. Mix a little more cheese (approx. 1 tbsp) with bread-crumbs. Sprinkle over top of casserole.
5. Bake at 350 degrees for at least 20 minutes.

Note: A great potluck dish, this recipe multiplies well. A deeper dish makes a moister product (more like a soufflé) and a shallower dish is a bit more like a crustless spinach pie. Serve hot or at room temperature. Leftovers reheat well.

**Reduced-fat mayo works fine, but not fat-free because the mayo is providing all the oil for the recipe.*

*****

Chicken and Rice Bake

(from Kim Rozsa, 2005 Conference Cookbook)

Ingredients:

1/4 cup	Reduced-fat margarine
1/3 cup	GF flour mix
3/4 tsp	Salt
1/8 tsp	Pepper

1-1/2 cup	Skim milk
1 cup	Chicken broth
2 cups	Cut-up chicken or turkey (about 10 oz.)
1-1/2 cup	Cooked white or wild rice
1/3 cup	Chopped green bell peppers
1/4 cup	Slivered almonds
2 tbsp	Chopped pimientos
4-oz can	Mushroom stems and pieces, drained
	Parsley, if desired

Directions:

1. Heat oven to 350 degrees.
2. Heat margarine in 2-qt saucepan over medium heat.
3. Stir in flour, sat and pepper.
4. Cook and stir constantly, until bubbly. Remove from heat.
5. Stir in milk and broth. Heat to boiling, stir constantly.
6. Boil and stir one minute.
7. Stir in remaining ingredients. Pour into greased 2-qt casserole or square 8 in. x 8 in. baking dish.
8. Bake uncovered 40–45 minutes or until bubbly. Garnish with parsley.

*****

Corn Tortilla Pizza

(from Mary Anderson, 2004 Conference Cookbook)

Ingredients:

2	Corn tortillas
	Sauce
	Toppings

Directions:

1. Put sauce between the tortillas to hold together.
2. Top with your favorite pizza toppings.
3. Bake 10–12 minutes.

Money-savingtTip: Instead of ready-made pizza shells use corn tortillas. One package of 10 will yield 5 small pizzas.

*****

Crunchy Chicken Nuggets

(from Jan Bowne, 1999 Conference Cookbook)

Ingredients:

2 whole	Chicken breasts, boneless, skinless, and cut into 1-1/2–2 in. cubes
1/4 cup	Rice flour
1/4 tsp.	Paprika
1/8 tsp.	Pepper
1	Egg, beaten
2 tbsp	Milk
1/2 cup	GF bread crumbs, toasted

Directions:

1. Combine flour, paprika, and pepper in large reclosable plastic bag.
2. Add chicken cubes, close, and shake to coat evenly.
3. In a small bowl combine egg and milk. Dip coated cubes into egg mixture.
4. In another reclosable plastic bag, place bread crumbs and add cubes to coat.
5. Place on baking sheet, bake at 400 degrees for 10–20 minutes.

*****

Eggplant Parmesan

(from Sherry Weinstein, 2004 Conference Cookbook)

Ingredients:

1 large	Eggplant
1 large	Egg, OR 2 egg whites

1 cup	Parmesan cheese
1/2 jar	Spaghetti sauce
1 cup	Shredded mozzarella cheese
3/4 tsp.	Dried basil
	Additional parmesan cheese for topping

Directions:

1. Cut eggplant lengthwise into 1/2-in. thick slices.
2. In pie plate, with fork beat egg with 1–2 tablespoons water until blended.
3. In another bowl, mix parmesan cheese and basil. Dip eggplant slices in egg mixture, then coat with parmesan mixture.
4. Arrange enough coated eggplant to fit in single layer on large cookie sheet.
5. Broil 10–12 minutes or until lightly browned on both sides, turning once.
6. Remove eggplant to plate. Repeat with remaining eggplant.
7. Change oven to 400 degrees.
8. In 9 in. x 13 in. baking dish, spoon some of the sauce and top with half of broiled eggplant, slightly overlapping.
9. Layer half of remaining sauce and half of the parmesan cheese. Repeat layering and sprinkle top with grated parmesan cheese.
10. Makes about 4 main servings.
11. Recipe can easily be doubled using 2 medium sized eggplants.

Note: This is a light version, since the eggplant is broiled instead of fried. The dish, which always wins raves, substitutes parmesan cheese for the bread crumbs.

*****

GF Lasagna

(from Mary Anderson, 2005 Conference Cookbook)

Ingredients:

1 lb	Ground beef, cooked and drained
1 jar	Your favorite GF spaghetti sauce or homemade sauce
6	GF lasagna noodles, cooked *al dente*
1	Egg, beaten
2 cups	Cottage cheese
1/2 cup	Grated parmesan cheese
8 oz.	Sliced mozzarella cheese
1 tbsp	Dried parsley flakes

Directions:

1. Combine egg, cottage cheese, 1/4 cup parmesan cheese and parsley flakes.
2. Combine ground beef and sauce.
3. Layer half of the cooked noodles in baking dish.
4. Spread half the cottage cheese mixture over noodles, then half the sauce mixture.
5. Top with half the mozzarella cheese. Repeat layers.
6. Sprinkle remaining parmesan cheese on top.

*****

Impossible Chicken 'n Broccoli Pie

(from Sylvia Bower, 2004 Conference Cookbook)

Ingredients:

10 oz.	Frozen chopped broccoli
3 cups	Shredded cheddar cheese
1-1/2 cups	Cooked chicken, cut up
2/3 cup	Chopped onion
1-1/3 cups	Milk
3	Eggs

3/4 cup	GF Bisquick mix
3/4 tsp.	Salt
1/4 tsp.	Pepper

Directions:

1. Heat oven to 400 degrees.
2. Grease 10 in. x 11 1/2 in. pie plate.
3. Rinse under running water to thaw. Drain thoroughly.
4. Mix broccoli, 2 cups cheese, chicken, and onions in pie plate.
5. Beat milk, eggs, baking mix, salt, and pepper until smooth—15 seconds in blender or 1 minute with hand mixer.
6. Pour into pie plate.
7. Bake 25–35 minutes, until knife inserted in center comes out clean.
8. Top with remaining cheese.
9. Bake 1–2 minutes longer, until cheese is melted.
10. Cool 5 minutes.
11. Make 6–8 servings.

*****

Jamaican Jerk Chicken

(from Bob Janosy, 2004 Conference Cookbook)

Ingredients:

6	Scallions, green only, sliced thin
2 large	Shallots, finely minced
2 large	Cloves garlic, finely minced
1 tbsp	Fresh ginger, finely minced
1 tsp.	Hot fresh chile (Scotch bonnet or habanero), seeded, finely chopped
1 tbsp	Ground allspice
1 tsp.	Fresh ground black pepper
1/4 tsp.	Cayenne pepper

1 tsp.	Ground cinnamon
1/2 tsp.	Ground nutmeg
1 tbsp	Fresh thyme or 1 tsp. dried
1 tsp.	Coarse salt
1 tbsp	Dark brown sugar
1/2 cup	Fresh orange juice
1/2 cup	Rice vinegar
1/4 cup	Red wine vinegar
1/4 cup	Soy sauce
1/4 cup	Olive oil
2	Chickens , quartered

Directions:

1. In small bowl, combine scallions, shallots, garlic, ginger, and chile.
2. In another bowl, combine spices, salt, and sugar. Mix thoroughly.
3. Whisk in orange juice, vinegars, and soy sauce.
4. Slowly drizzle in oil, whisking constantly.
5. Add reserved scallion mixture and stir. Let rest 1 hour.
6. Wash chicken and place in bowl.
7. Add sauce to chicken and rub in well (use gloves to protect hands from hot chiles).
8. Cover and refrigerate overnight.

*****

Polenta Lasagna

(from Denise Loehr, 2004 Conference Cookbook)

Ingredients:

1 tube	Polenta
	Cooking spray
15 oz.	Ricotta cheese
1/2 tsp.	Crushed red pepper
10 oz.	Frozen chopped spinach

2	Eggs, whites only
1 jar	Marinara sauce
1 cup	Parmesan cheese, fresh preshredded.

Directions:

1. Preheat oven to 400 degrees.
2. Spray 11 in. x 7 in. baking sheet with cooking spray.
3. Cut Polenta in 1/2-in. width and arrange on pan to from bottom layer.
4. Mix together ricotta cheese, red pepper, spinach, and egg. Spread over polenta.
5. Spoon marinara sauce on top evenly.
6. Cover with foil and bake for 30 minutes.
7. Uncover and sprinkle with cheese and bake for additional 5 minutes or until cheese melts.

*****

Skillet Enchiladas

(from Mary Louise McNamara, 2004 Conference Cookbook)

Ingredients:

1 lb.	Ground beef
1 medium	Onion, chopped
10 oz. can	GF enchilada sauce
1/3 cup	Milk
1–2 tbsp	Chopped green chilies, canned
	Oil
8	Corn tortillas
2-1/2 cups	Cheddar cheese, finely shredded, divided
1/2 cup	Ripe olives, chopped

Directions:

1. In a larger skillet, cook beef and onion over medium heat until meat is no longer pink. Drain.
2. Stir in sauce, milk, and chilies.

3. Bring to a boil. Reduce heat, cover, and simmer for 20 minutes. Stir occasionally.
4. Meanwhile in another skillet, heat 1/4-in. of oil.
5. Dip each tortilla in hot oil for 3 seconds on each side or just until limp. Drain on paper towels.
6. Top each with 1/4 cup cheese and 1 tablespoon olives.
7. Roll up and place over beef mixture, spooning some over enchiladas.
8. Cover and cook until heated through, about 15 minutes.
9. Sprinkle with remaining cheese, cover and cook until cheese is melted.

Money-saving tip: Instead of ready-made pizza shells use corn tortillas. One package of 10 will yield five small pizzas.

*****

Spinach Pie (Quiche)

(from Puri Purta, 2005 Conference Cookbook)

Ingredients:

10-oz. pkg	Frozen spinach
3	Eggs
12 oz	Cottage cheese
3 tbsp	Buckwheat flour
2 tbsp	Butter, melted
1 cup	Cheddar cheese, grated

Directions:

1. Preheat oven to 350 degrees.
2. Thaw spinach, squeeze out water, and chop.
3. Mix all the ingredients together.
4. Spray deep dish pie pan or square 9 in. x 9 in. pan with no-stick spray (Pam). Pour mixture.
5. Bake for 45 minutes to 1 hour until edges are brown.

*****

✓ *Sweet and Sour Pork*

(from Becky Paloci, 1999 Conference Cookbook)

Ingredients:

1-1/2 lb.	Pork, cut in cubes
2-lb. can	Pineapple chunks
1/4 cup	Brown sugar
2 tbsp	Cornstarch
1/4 cup	Cider vinegar
2–3 tbsp	GF soy sauce
1/2 tsp.	Salt
	Green pepper, strips
1/4 cup	Onion, thinly sliced

Directions:

1. Brown pork, add 1/2 cup water. Cover and simmer until tender, about 1 hour.
2. Drain pineapple and reserve juice.
3. Combine brown sugar, cornstarch, pineapple juice, vinegar, soy sauce, and salt.
4. Add to pork, cook, and stir until gravy thickens.
5. Add pineapple, green pepper, and onion.
6. Cook 2–3 minutes. Serve over rice.

Tip: This recipe was one my mother always made and it's wonderful! You also can use a pressure cooker for the pork or cook it in electric skillet or crock pot.

*****

SOUPS

Chinese Corn Soup

(from Karen Hutson, 2005 Conference Cookbook)

Ingredients:

2	Whole chicken breasts, boned and skinned
1	Egg white

1 tbsp	Rice wine
1 tbsp	Cornstarch
1 qt	Chicken stock
8 oz. can	Creamed corn
1 tsp	Salt
1-1/2 tsp	Pepper
1	Egg, beaten
2 tbsp	Cornstarch dissolved in 2 tbsp water

Directions:

1. Dice chicken into bite-sized pieced or slice to thin slivers and combine with the egg white, rice whine, and cornstarch. Set aside.
2. Bring to a boil the chicken stock, creamed corn, salt, and pepper.
3. When stock reached a boil, add chicken, stirring constantly to break up chicken. Cook 1 minute.
4. Add eggs in a thin stream, stirring slowly in one direction. Stir in cornstarch/water mixture. Cook 1–2 minutes.

Tip: If chicken stock is already salted, reduce salt in step #2.

*****

Susan's Potato Soup

(from Mary Louise McNamara, 2004 Conference Cookbook)

Ingredients:

4	Potatoes, peeled and chopped
1/4 cup	Celery, chopped
1/4 cup	Onion – chopped
1 tsp.	Parsley flakes
1 cube	Chicken bouillon (optional)
1/2 tsp.	Salt
11/2 cup	Milk
1/2 lb.	Velveeta, cubed

2 tbsp	GF Flour (optional)
	Pepper to taste

Directions:

1. In a large saucepan, bring to boil (with just enough water to cover) potatoes, celery, onion, parsley, bouillon cube, and seasonings.
2. Mix well, cover, and simmer until tender.
3. Mix milk and flour together and add to veggies.
4. Cook until thickened. Add cheese and stir until melted.
5. The cheese thickens the soup.

Note: Ham can be added!

*****

Tortilla Soup

(from Sandy Izsak, 2004 Conference Cookbook)

Ingredients:

6	6-in. corn tortillas
3 large	Tomatoes, chopped (3 cups)
4 medium	Carrots, sliced (2 cups)
1 large	Onion, chopped (1 cup)
1 cup	Water
14-1/2 oz. can	Chicken broth
4-1/2 oz. can	Chopped green chili peppers
2 tsp.	Chili powder
1/8 tsp.	Salt
15-oz. can	Pinto beans, rinsed and drained
1/3 cup	Snipped fresh cilantro
	Tabasco to taste (optional)

Directions:

1. Cut tortillas into 1/2-in. strips and cut in half crosswise.
2. Place on ungreased baking sheet. Bake 350 degrees for 10–13 minutes.

3. Set aside.
4. Combine all ingredients except for pinto beans and cilantro.
5. Bring to a boil, reduce heat, and simmer covered for 20 minutes.
6. Add beans and cilantro. Heat through.
7. Ladle soup into bowls. Divide strips among bowls.
8. Serve immediately.

*****

SALADS

Bean Salad

(from Carol Kimball, 2002 Conference Cookbook)

Ingredients:

1 can	Kidney beans
1 can	Wax beans
1 can	Green beans
1 medium	Onion, chopped
1	Green pepper, chopped
	Celery, chopped
1 cup	Vinegar
1 tbsp	Water
1/3 cup	Oil
1 cup	Sugar
1 tsp.	Salt
1 tsp.	Paprika

Directions:

1. Mix dressing well, coat beans, and serve chilled

*****

Broccoli Salad

(from Mary Anderson, 2005 Conference Cookbook)

Ingredients:

2 heads	Fresh broccoli
1/2	Sweet or red onion
1 cup	Shredded cheddar cheese
1 lb	Bacon
1 cup	Miracle Whip
1/2 cup	Sugar
2 tbsp	Apple cider vinegar

Directions:

1. Clean broccoli and chop into bite-sized pieces. Chop onion.
2. Fry bacon until crisp. Drain and crumble.
3. Mix broccoli, onion, bacon, and cheese.
4. Mix Miracle Whip, sugar, and vinegar. Mix into broccoli mix.
5. Can be topped with 1/4 cup raisins and/or nuts for more fiber.

*****

Cole Slaw

(from Terry Bradley, 2004 Conference Cookbook)

Ingredients:

16 oz.	Bag shredded cabbage and carrot cole slaw mix
12 oz.	Bag shredded broccoli, carrot and red cabbage slaw mix
1 to 1-1/2 cups	Mayonnaise (low-calorie or low-fat is fine)
3/4 cup	Sour cream (low-fat is fine)
3/4 cup	Apple cider vinegar
2 tsp.	Garlic powder

2 tsp.	Onion powder
1 tsp.	Salt (to taste)
1/2 tsp.	Pepper (to taste)

Directions:

1. Mix the dressing ingredients together in a large bowl.
2. Add the shredded vegetables and toss well to coat.
3. Keep mixture refrigerated until you're ready to serve.

*****

BREADS AND CRACKERS

Banana Nut Muffins

(from Jann Bowne)

Ingredients:

1/2 cup (1 stick)	Butter or margarine, softened
1 cup	Sugar
2 large	Eggs
2 large	Bananas, ripe, mashed
1 tsp	Vanilla
1 cup	Buttermilk
1/2 cup	Chopped pecans
2 cups	GF flour mix (part bean or sorghum flour)
1 tsp	Salt
1 tsp	Baking powder
1/2 tsp	Baking soda
1 tsp	Xanthan gum

Directions:

1. Preheat oven to 400. Grease (or line with muffin papers) 12 muffin pan cups.
2. Beat together butter and sugar at medium speed until light and fluffy.
3. Add eggs, one at a time, beating well after each addition. Beat in bananas until smooth.

4. Mix together dry ingredients.
5. Alternately stir flour mixture and buttermilk into egg mixture until dry ingredients are just moistened.
6. Stir in nuts and vanilla.
7. Spoon batter into prepared pan, filling half full. Bake until lightly golden, 15–18 minutes.
8. Remove from pan and cool on wire rack.

*****

Cheese Crackers

(from Barb Meek, 2004 Conference Cookbook)

Ingredients:

2 tbsp	Butter
1	Egg
1/2 tsp.	Salt
1/8 tsp.	Pepper
2 cups	Grated sharp cheddar cheese
3/4 cup	Rice flour
1/4 cup	Potato starch flour
1 tsp.	Xanthan gum
	Salt for sprinkling

Directions:

1. Preheat oven to 400 degrees.
2. In a mixer beat butter until creamy.
3. Add egg, salt, and pepper. Beat until blended.
4. Beat in the cheese until combined.
5. Separately mix the flours and xanthan gum. Add to cheese mixture.
6. Work dough into a ball. If needed to form a ball add one tablespoon of water at a time.
7. Don't worry about overworking. (My kids love to help. It is like playing with play dough!)
8. Divide ball in half and place on baking sheet. (or keep ball together and use a large airbake sheet).

9. Cover the ball with plastic wrap to roll out.
10. The thinner it is rolled out, the crunchier the cracker will be. The thicker it is rolled, the more it will taste like cheese bread.
11. When dough is spread out, sprinkle with salt and cut with pastry wheel. Make into 1-in. squares.
12. Bake 4–6 minutes until deep golden.

Note: Fiber can be added by adding 1–2 tsp. flax seed meal in step 5.

*****

Chocolate, Chocolate Chip Muffins

(from Beth Sisson, 2004 Conference Cookbook)

Note: This recipe is VERY high in calories, and it is great to bulk up calories in kids who are trying to gain weight. I also add flax seed meal to add fiber to their diet.

Ingredients:

1 stick	Butter or margarine
1-1/4 cups	Sugar
1	Egg
1-1/2 cup	Gluten-Free Pantry French Bread/ Pizza Mix
2-1/4 tsp.	Baking powder
1/8 tsp.	Salt
3/4–1 cup	Milk
1 tbsp	Flax seed meal (optional)
1/2 cup	Chocolate chips (optional)

Directions:

1. Mix butter and sugar until creamy. Add egg.
2. In a separate bowl, mix dry ingredients except chips.
3. Alternately add dry ingredients and milk to sugar mix.
4. Add chocolate chips.

5. Pour into muffin papers.
6. Bake at 350 degrees for 20–25 minutes if using regular-size papers.
7. Bake at 325 degrees for 15–20 minutes if using mini papers.

Note: The mini papers are a great way to get a picky little one to eat them!

*****

Graham Crackers

(from Barb Meek, 2004 Conference Cookbook)

Ingredients:

2 cups	Bette Hagman's Four Bean Flour Mix
1 tsp.	Xanthan gum
1-1/2 tsp.	Salt
1 tsp.	Cinnamon
2-1/2 tsp.	Baking powder
3/4 cup	Butter or margarine
1/4 cup	Honey
1 cup	Brown sugar
1 tsp.	Vanilla
1–2 tbsp	Water
	Cornstarch for rolling

Directions:

1. Whisk together dry ingredients and set aside.
2. In a large bowl beat remaining ingredients except water.
3. Add dry ingredients alternately with water, using just enough to hold the batter in a dough ball that will handle easily.
4. Refrigerate for at least one hour.
5. Preheat oven to 325 degrees.
6. Lightly grease two 12 in. x 15 in. baking sheets.

7. Using half the dough, work in some cornstarch if necessary to get a ball that isn't sticky.
8. Roll out on a cornstarch-dusted piece of plastic wrap to a rectangle 13 in. long.
9. Transfer to prepared baking sheet by placing a sheet over the dough and flipping the dough onto baking sheet.
10. Continue rolling out the dough until it completely covers the baking sheet and is about 1/8-in. thick.
11. Cut with pastry wheel.
12. Prick with a fork a couple of times.
13. Bake for about 30 minutes, removing crackers around the edge if they get too brown.

Note: Fiber can be added by adding 1–2 tsp. flax seed meal.

*****

Soft White Bread

(from Irene Edge, 2004 Conference Cookbook)

Ingredients:

Sift together:

2 cups	White rice flour
2 cups	Tapioca flour
4 tsp.	Xanthan gum
1/4 cup	Sugar
2/3 cup	Dry milk
1 tsp.	Salt

Stir in:

4 tsp.	Active dry yeast (2 packages)

Separately combine:

3	Eggs, beaten
2 cups	Water
4 tbsp	Margarine, melted
1 tsp.	Vinegar

Directions:

1. Mix all ingredients together.
2. Let dough rise in bowl.
3. Pour into greased bread pans and let dough rise.
4. Bake at 350 degrees for 20–25 minutes.

Tip: For pizza: Bake 12 minutes. Add toppings. Bake additional 15 minutes.

Potato Pizza: Bake crust. Melt 4 tsp. margarine, add 1/2 tsp. garlic. Spread over crust. Layer with sliced white potatoes (can be canned). Cover with Colby cheddar cheese. Sprinkle with bacon (cooked, cooled, and crumbled) and diced onions. Bake 15 minutes.

*****

West Tennessee Corn Bread

(from Brenda Lucas, 2002 Conference Cookbook)

Ingredients:

1	Egg
1/4 cup	Mayonnaise (do NOT use reduced-fat or fat-free)
1/4 cup	Buttermilk
1 tbsp	Oil
1 cup	Yellow cornmeal
1/4 cup	Sugar
1-1/2 tsp.	Baking powder
1/4 tsp.	Salt

Directions:

1. In bowl, beat first four ingredients until smooth.
2. Combine remaining ingredients and add to egg mixture.
3. Place in greased and dusted (with cornmeal) ovenproof 6-in. skillet or round baking dish.
4. Bake 425 degrees for 18–20 minutes.

*****

Cookies and Desserts

Buckeyes in Winter

(from Sylvia Bower)

Dough

1 1/2 cups	GF flour
1 tsp.	Xanthun gum
1/2 tsp.	Salt
1/2 cup	Unsweetened cocoa
1/2 tsp.	Baking soda
1/2 cup	White sugar
1/2 cup	Brown sugar
1/2 cup	Butter (one stick)
1/4 cup	Creamy peanut butter
1 tsp.	Vanilla
1	Egg

Filling

3/4 cup	Creamy peanut butter
3/4 cup	Powdered sugar

Instructions:

1. Preheat oven to 375 degrees.
2. In a small bowl combine flour, xanthun gum, salt, cocoa, and baking soda. Blend well and set aside. (Or mix in a tightly sealed plastic bag.)
3. In a large mixing bowl, beat the sugars, butter, and peanut butter until light and fluffy.
4. Add vanilla and egg, beating well.
5. Stir in flour mixture until blended. Refrigerate while making filling.
6. In a small bowl, combine peanut butter and powdered sugar and blend well.
7. Using your hands, form twenty 1- to 2-in. balls of the filling (they expand while baking).

8. To make the Buckeyes, shape one teaspoon of dough into a round flat patty.
9. Place a filling ball in the center and ease the dough around it, covering it, but leaving a small opening to resemble a buckeye.
10. Bake at 375 deggrees for 7–9 minutes until set.
11. Remove immediately and roll in powdered sugar.

Yield-: About 20 cookies.

*****

Deluxe Buckwheat Almond Cake

(from Sherry Weinstein; reprinted with permission from The Birkett Mills Buckwheat Cookbook, The Birkett Mills, Penn Yan, NY)

Ingredients:

1- 1/2 cups	Sliced almonds, with skin on
3/4 cup	Unsalted butter, softened
3/4 cup	Sugar, divided
4	Eggs, separated
1/8 tsp.	Salt
2 tsp.	Vanilla extract
1/2 cup	Light buckwheat flour
1/2 cup	Raspberry preserves
	10-in. round paper doily
1 tbsp	Confectioners' sugar

Instructions:

1. Oil bottom of 9 in. x 1-1/2 in. round cake pan and line with waxed paper.
2. Finely grind almonds in food processor, blender, or nut-chopper.
3. In large bowl, cream butter and 6 tablespoons sugar. Beat in yolks, one at a time. Stir in vanilla and almonds.

4. In medium bowl, beat egg whites and salt to soft peaks; gradually add remaining sugar, beating until soft, glossy peaks form.
5. Lightly fold one-fourth of the beaten whites into the batter. Sift one-fourth of the flour over batter; combine lightly. Alternately add remaining whites and flour in this manner.
6. Pour batter into pan. Bake at 350 degrees for 30 minutes or until tester inserted into center comes out clean.
7. Cool on rack 10 minutes; remove from pan.
8. When cool, slice horizontally into two layers. Place bottom layer, cut side up, on plate; spread with preserves. Top with remaining layer, cut side down.
9. Place doily on top; sprinkle with confectioner's sugar; remove doily.

*****

Easy Flourless Chocolate Cake

(from Sylvia Bower)

Ingredients:

1/2 cup	Unsalted butter
3/4 cup	Sugar
3	Eggs
4 oz.	Bittersweet chocolate
1/2 cup	Unsweetened cocoa
	Ganache (*recipe follows*)
	Whipped cream

Preheat oven to 375 degrees. Grease an 8-in. round pan.

In a double boiler over barely simmering water, melt chocolate and butter until smooth. Remove from heat and whisk in sugar. Add eggs and combine well. Sift in cocoa powder and whisk until smooth. Pour batter into prepared pan. Bake for about 25 minutes or until thin crust is formed.

Cool cake for 5 minutes before removing from pan to cool completely on rack. Transfer to serving plate and dust lightly with cocoa powder or spread with ganache. Refrigerate.

Ganache

1/4 cup	Heavy cream
2 tbsp	Unsalted butter
4 oz.	Semisweet chocolate, chopped or chips

In a small pan, bring the cream and butter to a boil. Remove from heat, add chocolate and stir until smooth.

*****

Easy Fruit Salad

(from Diane Lott)

Ingredients:

1 can	Lite chunky mixed fruit
1 can	Pineapple tidbits or chunks in natural juice
1 pkg (12–16 oz)	Frozen strawberries, thawed
2	Bananas, sliced

Chill canned fruit. Mix together with thawed strawberries and bananas. Served chilled.

*****

Fruit Fluff

(from Stephanie Olson, 2004 Conference Cookbook)

Ingredients:

8 oz.	Cool Whip
1 pkg.	Kroger (GF) Vanilla Pudding, small
3/4 cup	Milk (or soy milk)
1 can	Mandarin oranges, drained
2	Bananas, sliced

Directions:

1. Whip together the Cool Whip, pudding, and milk together for a base.
2. Fold in the fruit.

Tip: Any fruits can be substituted for the bananas and oranges. Try strawberries, grapes, pineapple, or any other that "tickles your fancy."

*****

Million Dollar Salad

(from Elizabeth Sager, 2002 Conference Cookbook)

Ingredients:

1 can	Sweetened condensed milk
1/2 cup	Lemon juice
20 oz. can	Crushed pineapple, well-drained
1 cup	Coconut
1 cup	Chopped pecans
1 large tub	Cool Whip

Directions:

1. Combine milk with lemon juice; add remaining ingredients. Delicious!

CHAPTER 14

Resources

by Mary Kay Sharrett

General

Gluten-Free Diet: A Comprehensive Resource Guide
by Shelley Case
Regina, SK, Canada: Case Nutritional Consulting, 2004
www.glutenfreediet.ca

Kids with Celiac Disease: A Family Guide to Raising Happy, Healthy, Gluten-Free Children
by Danna Korn
Bethseda, MD: Woodbine House (2001)
www.woodbinehouse.com

Wheat-Free, Worry-Free: The Art of Healthy Happy Gluten-Free Living
by Danna Korn
Carlsbad, CA: Hay House, 2002

Eating Gluten-Free with Emily
by Bonnie J. Kruszka; Illustrated by Richard S. Cihlar
Bethesda, MD: Woodbine House, 2004
www.woodbinehouse.com

Gluten-Free Friends: An Activity Book for Kids
by Nancy Patin-Falini
Littleton, CO: Savory Palate, Inc., 2004
www.savorypalate.com

Celiac Disease Nutrition Guide
by Tricia Thompson and Merri Lou Dobler
Chicago, IL: American Dietetic Association, 2003
www.eatright.org

Cook Books

Wheat-Free, Gluten-Free: 200 Delicious Dishes To Make Eating a Pleasure
by Michelle Berriedale-Johnson
Chicago, IL: Surrey Books, 2002

Nothing Beats Gluten-Free Cooking: A Children's Cookbook
edited by Anne Roland Lee, Laura Leon, and Susan Cohen
New York: Celiac Disease Center at Columbia University
www.celiacdiseasecenter.columbia.edu

Gluten Free 101 (2003)
Special Diet Solutions (1997)
Wheat-Free Recipes & Menus (1995)
Special Diet Celebrations (1999)
by Carol Fenster, Ph.D.
Littleton, CO: Savory Palate, Inc.
www.savorypalate.com

The Gluten-Free Gourmet: Living Well Without Wheat, Second Edition (2000)
More From The Gluten-Free Gourmet: Delicious Dining Without Wheat (1993)

The Gluten-Free Gourmet Cooks Fast and Healthy: Wheat-Free and Gluten-Free with Less Fuss and Less Fat (2000)
The Gluten-Free Gourmet Bakes Bread: More Than 200 Wheat-Free Recipes (2000)
The Gluten-Free Gourmet Makes Dessert (2002)
The Gluten-Free Gourmet Cooks Comfort Foods: Creating Old Favorites with the New Flours (2004)
by Bette Hagman
New York: Henry Holt and Company, Inc.

The Wheat-Free Gluten-Free Reduced Calorie Cookbook
Wheat-Free Gluten-Free Cookbook for Special Diets
www.homestead.com/gfkids/gf.html

Gluten-Free Baking
by Rebecca Reilly
New York: Simon and Schuster, 2002

Delicious Gluten-Free, Wheat-Free Breads
by LynnRae Ries
Phoenix, AZ: What? No Wheat? Enterprises
www.whatnowheat.com

Cooking Gluten-Free
by Karen Robertson
Celiacpublishing@earthlink.net

The Gluten-Free Kitchen: Over 135 Delicious Recipes for People with Gluten Intolerance or Wheat Allergy
by Roben Ryberg
New York: Three Rivers Press, 2000
www.primapublishing.com

Incredible Edible Gluten-Free Food for Kids
by Sheri L Sanderson
Bethesda, MD: Woodbine House, 2002
www.woodbinehouse.com

The Wheat-Free Gluten-Free Dessert Cookbook
Wheat-Free Gluten-Free Cookbook for Kids & Busy Adults
by Connie Sarros
Chicago, IL: Contemporary Books, 2004

Food Allergy Field Guide
by Theresa Willingham
Littleton, CO: Savory Palate, Inc.
www.savorypalate.com

Magazines

Bob and Ruth's Dining and Travel Club
www.bobandruths.com

Gluten-Free Living
edited and published by Ann Whelan
www.glutenfreeliving.com

Living Without
www.livingwithout.com

Scott Free Newsletter
edited by Scott Adams
www.celiac.com

Shopping Guides

Clan Thompson
Shopping Guide Data Base for a PC and Palm OS
Pocket Shopping Guide
www.clanthompson.com

Tri-County Celiac Support Group Shopping Guide and Newsletter
www.tccsg.com

Internet

Celiac Discussion List Archives
http://listserv.icors.org/archives/celiac.html

R.O.C.K (Raising Our Celiac Kids Web site)
www.celiackids.com

General Information

American Celiac Disease Alliance
www.americanceliac.org

Celiac Organization
www.celiac.com

Center for Celiac Research
www.celiaccenter.org

Gluten Freeda
www.glutenfreeda.com

National Digestive Diseases Clearinghouse
www.niddk.nih.gov/health/digest/pubs/celiac/index.htm

National Institute of Health Consensus Conference on Celiac Disease
http://consensus.nih.gov/cons/118/118cdc_intro.htm

Steve Plogsted Pharm.D Medication list
www.glutenfreedrugs.com

University of Chicago
www.uchospitals.edu/areas/pediatrics/celiac-disease

National Resource Groups

Canadian Celiac Association
www.celiac.ca
Ph: (905) 507-6208

Celiac Disease Foundation
www.celiac.org
Ph: (818) 990-2354

Celiac Sprue Association, United States of America
www.csaceliacs.org
Ph. (402) 558-0600

The Gluten Intolerance Group (GIG)
www.gluten.net
Ph.(206) 246-6552

Gluten-Free Companies

1-2-3 Gluten-Free, Inc.
www.123glutenfree.com

Amazing Grains (Montina™)
www.amazinggrains.com

Amy's Kitchen
www.amyskitchen.com

Authentic Foods
www.authenticfoods.com

Bob's Red Mill Natural Foods, Inc.
www.bobsredmill.com

Chebe Bread
www.chebe.com

Econatural Solutions/The Ruby Range
www.therubyrange.com El

Edwards and Sons Trading Company, Inc.
www.edwardsandsons.com

Ener-G Foods, Inc.
www.ener-g.com

Enjoy Life Foods
www.enjoylifefoods.com

Food For Life Baking Company
www.food-for-life.com

Garden Spot Distributors
www.gardenspotdist.com

Gifts of Nature
www.giftsofnature.com

The Gluten-Free Mall
www.glutenfreemall.com

Gluten-Free Pantry
www.glutenfree.com

The Gluten-Free Trading Company
www.glutenfree.net

Gluten Solutions
www.glutensolutions.com

Kingsmill Food
www.kingsmillfoods.com

Kinnikinnick Foods, Inc
www.kinnikinnick.com

Manna From Anna
www.glutenevolution.com

Maple Grove Foods
www.maplegrovefoods.com

Masuya (USA), Inc.
www.masuyanaturally.com

Mrs. Leepers
www.mrsleepers.com

Nature's Path
www.naturespath.com

Nu-World Amaranth
www.nuworldfoods.com

Pamela's Products
www.pamelasproducts.com

Peto Product, Ltd.
www.elpeto.com

Rizopia Food Products, Inc.
www.rizopia.com

Sylvan Border farms
www.sylvanborder.com

Tinkyada
www.tinkyada.com

Vans International Foods
www.vanswaffles.com

Bibliography

Addolorato G; Diguida D; De Rossi G; Valenza V; Domenicali M; Caputo F; Gasbarrini A; Capristo E; Gasbarrini G. "Regional cerebral hypoperfusion in patients with celiac disease," *American Journal of Medicine*, 2004 Mar 1; Vol. 116 (5), pp. 312-317.

Addolorato G; Capristo E; Ghittoni G; Valeri C; Masciana R; Ancona C; Gasbarrini G. "Anxiety but not depression decreases in coeliac patients after one-year gluten-free diet: a longitudinal study." *Scandinavian Journal of Gastroenterology*, 2001 May; Vol. 36 (5), pp. 502-506.

Agardh D; Nilsson A; Tuomi T; Linberg B; Carlsson AK; Lernmark A; Ivarsson SA. "Prediction of silent celiac disease at diagnosis of childhood type I diabetes by tissue transglutaminase autoantibodies and HLA." *Pediatric Diabetes*. 2001 Jun 2; (2): pp. 58-65.

American Osteopathic College of Dermatology: Dermatological Disease Database http://www.aocd.org/skin/dermatologic_diseases/dermatitis_herpeti.html

Bizzaro N; Villalta D; Tonutti E; Tampoia M; Bassetti D; Tozzoli R. "Association of celiac disease with connective tissue diseases and autoimmune diseases of the digestive tract." *Autoimmunity Reviews*, 2003 Oct. Vol. 2 (6), pp. 358-363.

Book L; Hart A; Black J; Feolo M; Zone JJ; Neuhausen SL. "Prevalence and clinical characteristics of celiac disease in Downs syndrome in a US study." *American Journal of Medical Genetics*, 2001 Jan 1; Vol. 98 (1), pp. 70-74.

Bushara KO, "Neurological presentation of celiac disease." *Gastroenterology*, 2005 Apr; Vol. 128 (4 Suppl1), pp. S92-97.

Carta MG; Hardoy MC; Usai P; Carpiniello B; Angst J. "Recurrent brief depression in celiac disease." *Journal of Psychosomatic Res*. 2003 Dec; 55 (6), pp. 573-574.

Carta MG; Hardoy MC; Boi MF; Mariotti S; Carpiniello B; Usai P. "Association between panic disorder, major depressive disorder, and celiac disease: possible role of thyroid autoimmunity." *Journal Psychosomatic Res*. 2002 Sep; 53 (3), pp. 789-793.

Ciacca C; Iavarone A; Siniscalchi M; Romano R; DeRosa A. "Psychological dimensions of celiac disease: toward an integrated approach." *Digetive Disease Sci*. 2002 Sep; 47 (9), pp. 2082-2087.

Duggan JM. "Coeliac disease: the great imitator." *Medical Journal of Australia*, 2004 May 17; 180 (10), pp. 524-526.

Eliakim R; Sherer DM. "Celiac disease: fertility and pregnancy." *Gynecol Obstet Invest*. 2001; 51 (1), pp. 3-7.

Fasano A; Berti I; Gerarduzzi T; Not T; Colletti RB; Drago S; Elitsur Y; Green P; Guandalini S; Hill ID; Pietzak M; Ventura A; Thorpe M; Kryszak D; Fornaroli F; Wasserman SS; Murray JA; Horvath K. "Prevalence of celiac disease in at-risk and not-at risk groups in the United States: a large multicenter study." Center for Celiac Research, University of Maryland School of Medicine, 22 S. Greene St. N5W70, PO Box 140, Baltimore, MD 21201-1595.

Fasano A. "Celiac disease finally moves to primetime in the United States," *Medscape*, October 14, 2003.

Fenster C. *Gluten-Free 101 Easy Basic Dishes Without Wheat*, Savory Palate, Inc., 8174 South Holly, #404 Centennial CO. 80122-4004. Copyright 2003.

Freeman HJ. "Strongly positive tissue transglutaminase antibody assays without celiac disease." *Canadian Journal of Gastroenterology* 2004 Jan; Vol 18 (1), pp. 25-28.

Green MD, Peter. *Celiac Disease: A Hidden Epidemic*, Collins, New York, 2005.

Green, PH; Jabri B. "Celiac disease and other precursors to small-bowel malignancy." *Gastroenterology Clinics of North America*, 2002 Jun; Vol. 31 (2), pp. 625-639.

Green PH, Jabri B. "Celiac disease." *Lancet* 2003 Aug 2; 362 (9381), pp. 383-391.

Green, PH; Rostami K; Marsh MN. "Diagnosis of coeliac disease." *Best Practice and Research Clinical Gastroenterology,* 2005 Jun; Vol. 19 (3), pp. 389-400.

Green PH; Pampertab SD. "Small bowel carcinoma and celiac disease." *Gut* 2004 May; Vol 53 (5), p. 774.

Gudjonsdotter AH; Nilsson S; Ek J; Kristiansson B; Ascher H. "The risk of celiac disease in 107 families with at least two affected siblings." *Journal of Pediatric Gastroenterology Nutrition*, 2004 Mar; 38 (3), pp. 338-342.

Hagman B. *The Gluten-Free Gourmet: Living Well Without Wheat*. Owl Books, New York, 2000.

Haskinson S; Colditz G; Manson J; Speizer F; editors. *Healthy Women, Healthy Lives: A Guide to Preventing Disease, from the Landmark Nurses, Health Study*. Simon and Schuster, New York, 2001.

Hoffenberg EJ; MacKenzie T; Barriga KJ; Eisenbarth GS; Bao F; Haas JE; Erlich H; Bugawan TI T; Sokol RJ; Taki I; Norris JM. "A prospective study of the incidence of childhood celiac disease." *Journal of Pediatrics* 2003 Sep; 143 (3), pp. 308-314.

Howdle PD; Holmes GK. "Small bowel malignancy in coeliac disease. *Gut* 2003 Aug; 52 (8), pp. 1211-1214.

Leffler D; Saha S; Farrell RJ. "Celiac disease." *The American Journal of Managed Care*." 2003 Dec; Vol. 9 (12), pp. 825-831.

Lepers S; Couignoux S; Colombel JF; Dubucquoi S. "Celiac disease in adults: new aspects." *La Revue de medicine interne*. 2004 Jan; Vol. 25 (1), pp. 22-34.

Matthews, DA. *The Faith Factor: Proof of the Healing Power of Prayer*. Penguin, New York, 1998.

Merck Manual of Diagnosis and Therapy, www.merck.com, Section 10, Chap. 120.

Murray JA; Watson T; Clearman B; Mitros F. "Effect of a gluten-free diest on gastrointestinal symptoms in celiac disease." *American Journal of Clinical Nutrition*, 2004 April; Vol. 79 (4), pp. 669-673.

Moreno ML; Vazquez H; Mazure R; Smecuol E; Niveloni S; Pedreire S; Sugai E; Maurino E; Gomez JC; Bai JC. "Stratification of bone fracture risk in patients with celiac disease." *Clinical Gastroenterology/Hepatology*, 2004 Feb; 2 (2), pp. 127-134.

National Institutes of Health, National Institute of Diabetes and Digestive and Kidney Diseases, Celiac Disease. www.digestive.niddk.nih.gov/diseases/pubs/celiac.

Petroniene R; Dubcenco E; Baker JP; Ottaway CA; Tang SJ; Zanati SA; Streutker CJ; Gardiner GW; Warren RE; Jeejeebhoy KN. "Given capsule endoscopy in celiac disease." *American Journal Gastroenterology* 2005 Mar; Vol. 100 (3), pp. 685-694.

Potocki P; Hozyasz K. "Psychiatric symptoms and coeliac disease." *Psychiatria polska [Psychiatr Pol]*, 2002 Jul–Aug; Vol. 36 (4), pp. 567-578.

Rostami K; Steegers EA; Wong WY; Braat DD; Steegers-Theunissen RP. "Coeliac disease and reproductive disorders: a neglected association." *European Journal of Obstetrics and Gynocology and Reproductive Biology*. 2001 Jun; Vol. 96 (2), pp. 146-149.

Sanchez-Albisua I; Wolf J; Neu A; Geiger H; Wascher I; Stern M. "Coeliac disease in children with type I diabetes mellitus: the effect of the gluten-free diet." *Diabetes Medicine*, 2005 Aug; Vol. 22 (8), pp. 1079-1082.

Siegel S. *Prescriptions for Living* HarperCollins, New York, 1998.

Silink M. M.D. "How should we manage celiac disease in childhood diabetes?" *Pediatric Diabetes*, 2001 Jun; 2 (2), pp. 58-65.

"The New Medicine," PBS Documentary, shown April 6, 2006. Directed by Muffie Meyer.

Whalen A. *Gluten-Free Living*, Vol. 9, No. 2. Ann Whalen, editor and publisher, 19A Broadway, Hawthorne, NY 10532.

Zebrowska A, Narbutt J, Sysa-Jedrzejowska A, Kobos J, Waszczkowska E. The imbalance between mettallo-proteinases and their tissue inhibitors is involved in the pathogenesis of dermatitis herpetiformis. *Mediators of Inflammation*. 2005 Dec: 2005(6), 373-379.

Glossary

Anemia Reduction below normal in the number of red cells or quantity of hemoglobin that occurs when (1) blood production is disturbed, (2) blood loss, (3) poor or lack of iron absorption.

Antibodies Cells that the body develops when it feels it is being attacked (simplified definition). Wikipedia definition: An **antibody** is a protein used by the immune system to identify and neutralize foreign objects like bacteria and viruses. Each antibody recognizes a specific antigen unique to its target. Production of antibodies is referred to as the_humoral immune system.

Aphthous stomatitis Sores in the oral mucosa commonly called canker sores. (Not caused by the herpes simplex virus.)

Arrhythmia Abnormal heart rate.

Celiac/coeliac disease Also referred to as celiac sprue, gluten-sensitive enteropathy, and nontropical sprue. Symptoms include one or more of the following: gas, abdominal pain, bloating, chronic diarrhea, pale foul-smelling stools, weight loss/weight gain, fatigue, anemia, bone or joint pain, osteoporosis/osteopenia, behavioral changes, tingling numbness in legs, muscle cramps, seizures, missed menstrual periods, infertility, recurrent miscarriage, delayed growth (children), failure to thrive (infants), aphthous ulcers (sores in the mouth).

Constipation Infrequent or difficult evacuation of feces (stool).

Crohn's disease An inflammation of the digestive tract. Most commonly affects the lower part of the small intestine called the ilium. The swelling extends deep into the lining of the affected area (all layers may be involved). Also called ileitis or enteritis. Symptoms include: abdominal pain, diarrhea, bloating, weight loss and/or bleeding.

Dental enamel hypoplasia Loss of enamel on teeth due to malabsorption of calcium.

Dermatitis herpetiformis Skin condition that occurs in 25% of CD patients. The skin eruptions are extremely itchy and are a manifestation of the damage that is happening in the small intestine.

Diabetes mellitus type I Usually called juvenile diabetes which is a condition requiring insulin to regulate the blood sugar.

Diabetes mellitus type II Common onset is over 40 years of age. Controlled with hypoglycemic medication and diet.

Diarrhea Abnormal and frequent liquid evacuation of feces (stool).

Down syndrome A chromosomal condition associated with mental retardation, characteristic facial expressions, and poor muscle tone. Increased risk of other physical conditions.

Endomysial antibodies Antibodies produced when the gluten in grains are introduced into an individual with CD.

Endoscopy Procedure that allows the gastroenterologist to examine and biopsy the esophagus, stomach, duodenum, and small intestine by using a tube (scope) with a light on it.

Enriched Adding back nutrients lost during the processing of the food product.

Fortified Adding nutrients that are not present in the original product.

Gluten-free diet A diet that contains no known proteins of wheat, barley, and/or rye. (2008 FDA is required to identify a description of gluten-free.)

Gluten-sensitive enteropathy A diagnosis frequently used for CD.

Hemoglobin An iron-containing red blood cell that functions to transport oxygen from the lungs to the tissues of the body.

Hordein A protein complex found in barley that produces antibodies in an individual with CD.

Hypochondria (hypochondriac) Severe anxiety about one's health associated with numerous and varying symptoms that cannot be attributed to disease.

Iron deficiency anemia Caused by iron deficiency either by blood loss, malabsorption of iron in the small intestine, or disturbance of blood production.

Irritable bowel syndrome An inflammation of the intestine that can occur in any part of the intestinal tract from various causes. Symptoms include: diarrhea, abdominal bloating, abdominal pain, and constipation.

Lactose intolerance Inability to digest lactose, which is the sugar found in milk. Results in abdominal pain, bloating, gas, and possible diarrhea.

Lupus erythematosis (SLE) Autoimmune disease that is a generalized connective tissue disorder, usually involving several body systems.

Malabsorption Any condition that prevents nutrients from being absorbed from foods into the digestive tract.

Multiple sclerosis A disease in which there are lesions in the central nervous system causing numbness, speech problems, and visual problems. It has periods of remission and is a long-term condition.

Multisystem disorder More than one system in the body is affected. In CD, the gastrointestinal tract is involved; however, the skin, brain, and other areas of the body may be involved.

Osteoporosis Calcium deficiency that results in bones becoming porous and increasing a risk of fracture.

Peripheral neuropathy Loss of feeling in the fingers or toes as a result of nerve endings dying.

Prolamines A protein complex found in grains that produces antibodies in an individual with CD.

Seculin A protein complex found in rye that produces antibodies in an individual with CD.

Sjogren's syndrome Autoimmune disease that occurs in middle aged or older women. Symptoms include: dryness of the mouth, inflammation of the eyes, and enlargement of the parotid glands.

Small intestine The area of the digestive tract between the stomach and large intestine. It contains the villi (or folds) which absorb most nutrients.

Sprue A term formerly used for celiac disease (celiac sprue).

Turner syndrome Chromosomal condition that affects development in females.

Ulcerative colitis Inflammation and sores in lining of the rectum and colon. Symptoms include: diarrhea, abdominal pain, anemia, fatigue, loss of appetite, weight loss, rectal bleeding, skin lesions, joint pain, and growth failure (children).

Villi The small hair-like projections in the small intestine that absorb nutrients from food.

Williams syndrome Developmental disorder that affects many parts of the body. Mild to moderate mental retardation, unique personal characteristics, distinctive facial features, and heart and blood vessel problems.

Wireless capsule endoscopy A minuturized camera that is swallowed and remotely visualizes the intestinal tract.

Xanthun gum Substance added to gluten-free baked products to add elasticity to the dough.

Index